THE THREE RULES

To Lose Weight And Keep
It Off Forever

By Harold Oster, MD

To Angie and Troy, the best people I know.
And to Ryan Holiday, whose books changed my life.

TABLE OF CONTENTS

Preface: How I Discovered the Rules

It took me three decades, but I figured it out.

I excel at losing weight. I am better at gaining it. The Three Rules is not a scheme to lose weight quickly, it will help you lose weight and keep it off forever. This book is for people like me, people willing to work hard at something important. Losing weight is hard and keeping it off is hard. But you can do it. *The Three Rules to Lose Weight and Keep It Off Forever* will help you.

My approach to self-improvement has changed over my life, and now I am trying to live the values of the Stoics, who lived around 2000 years ago. If you know little about Stoicism, it is not what you have imagined. It does not teach us to be unemotional and hard-hearted. It teaches us how to live the best life we can. There are many sources, and my first real exposure to Stoicism was when I read *The Obstacle Is The Way* by Ryan Holiday.[1] Holiday teaches that we become better by confronting and overcoming obstacles. *The Three Rules to Lose Weight And Keep It Off Forever* embraces the same philosophy. Anyone can overcome the obstacle of weight control by following The Rules in this book. It is hard; it is an obstacle, but you can overcome it. You will be better for it.

I am working to become healthier and to stay healthy for as long as possible. The most important step has been to lose weight and keep it off. In medical school, we did not learn much about obesity. It was nowhere near as common as it is now, though we saw obese patients. Obesity was just not an important topic. We learned about obesity-related

---

[1] Holiday, Ryan. *The Obstacle Is The Way: The Timeless Art of Turning Trials Into Triumph.* New York: Portfolio/Penguin, 2014.

illnesses, such as diabetes and heart failure, but the professors did not stress the causes and treatments of obesity. They taught us that if you ate too much, you would gain weight. If you cut back and exercised, you would lose weight. That is true, as far as it goes. But why do so many people struggle? Why is obesity becoming more and more common, if everyone knows why we gain weight, and everyone knows how to lose it?

When I was very young, I thought doctors were doctors, pilots were pilots, and plumbers were plumbers. They were not regular people. Now I know that everyone in every profession has their own life, and even doctors can be overweight or thin, healthy or sick. My struggle was always my weight and control over my eating. I gained and lost weight many times over many years, and many of my patients were struggling in the same way. Over time, I developed various strategies for my patients and for myself. I have settled on the Three Rules as the best strategy for most people. What I did not learn in medical school, I learned in my life and in the office with my patients.

Losing weight has so many benefits. You will feel better, have more opportunities to enjoy life, and be healthier. Yes, it is hard to lose weight. If it were easy, there would not be an obesity problem, and there would be no demand for books like this. Anyone that tells you otherwise is wrong or lying. As the saying goes, nothing worth doing is easy.

Some health problems require medications or surgery, just as some projects at home require an expert. There is a role for medical intervention in weight management, but only if you have tried everything first. You can lose weight and keep it off on your own, if you work hard enough. I do not believe the clichés that anyone can do absolutely anything they set out to do if they work hard. I could never play NBA basketball or become a chess grandmaster. But I believe anyone can lose weight. It is hard. Do it anyway.

I Know How to Lose Weight

I had a good childhood. I was healthy, half-way athletic, and ate well. I was never obese, but I was consistently up a few pounds, and I was never as lean as my brother. A few times in high school, I tried to lose some weight and was somewhat successful. Too many lunches at Burger King with my best friend always led to a rapid return to my previous weight. In my first year of medical school at the University of Miami, I stress-ate and realized I was about 20 pounds overweight, on my five-foot, five-inch frame. I started a diet.

This first real diet was low-calorie. Low-calorie diets are typically low fat, since fat has more calories per gram than anything else. I ate mostly salads at Burger King and small meals at home. A snack was a piece of bread, sometimes toasted. I did not enjoy it and was hungry most of the time. But it worked, and I lost the weight. The following year, I was heavy again, largely from the wonderful chicken sandwich and fries at Wendy's, conveniently near the University of Miami library. A few months later, I dieted again with calorie-cutting, was again hungry most of the time, and lost another 20 pounds. I kept track of my weight in a little green note-book, in which I also recorded interesting medical facts, formulas, and phone numbers. Over the next several years, I gained weight and then dieted, always with the same hunger. But it always worked because I was disciplined. It was stressful; I was always hungry, but it worked.

In 1996, I was about 25 pounds overweight, and I was about to start a very difficult rotation of my fellowship training in Infectious Diseases at Mount Sinai Hospital in Miami Beach. I wanted to lose weight, but I knew I would have difficulty being hungry during stressful, long days. Then I learned of *Dr. Atkins New Diet Revolution*.[2] Robert Atkins did not invent the low-carbohydrate diet, but he brought it to the public attention. He believed that cutting out virtually all carbohydrates leads to weight loss without hunger. He was right. The diet works, and there are few health risks of the diet, at least in the short term.

Over the next 6 weeks, I got to the hospital cafeteria very early, where I ate breakfast and planned my long day of seeing patients. I ate omelets, sausage, and ham. I saw patients all morning and had lunch: cheeseburgers without the bun, chicken salad, tuna salad, eggs, cheese and anything low in carbohydrates and high in protein and fat. I worked through the afternoon and evening, regularly arriving home after 8PM. I ate steak,

---

[2] Atkins, Robert C. *Dr. Atkins' New Diet Revolution.* New York: Quill, 2002.

fried Spam (my favorite) and more eggs and cheese. I lost 25 pounds in six weeks. And I was never hungry.

After the rotation was over, I felt that I could just eat sensibly, in moderation. I did fine for a while, but then I resumed my old habits—snacks, breads, some fast food. In less than 6 months, I was again 20 pounds overweight. I have since misplaced my green notebook with the details, but I gained and lost weight multiple times over the next six or eight years. Mostly, I did the Atkins Diet, because giving up carbohydrates (from now on I will usually say carbs) while eating more protein and fat was easier for me than hunger. But every time, after I completed the diet, thinking I could just eat my usual food in moderation, I gained the weight back. I did not realize the obvious. I could not eat sensibly. I could not eat junk food and carbs in moderation.

What ended my use of the Atkins Diet is not an issue for most people. Worried about the health effects, I had my cholesterol checked. Healthy total cholesterol being under 200, mine was over 475 and my LDL, the so-called bad cholesterol, was about 400. I had it repeated and confirmed. I even spoke to an expert on the effects of the Atkins Diet. He said that this rise in cholesterol was uncommon, and he asked me to stay on the diet and have my blood sent to him to determine if I was a hyper-absorber of cholesterol. I told him to forget it, not wanting another day of a cholesterol level that high. I have confirmed in reading and with my patients that most people do not have a significant rise in cholesterol on the diet.

After a few more times gaining and losing weight (back exclusively to calorie-cutting and hunger), I was frustrated. At about that time, The *South Beach Diet*,[3] by Arthur Agatston, MD (from the same hospital where I first tried the Atkins Diet) became popular. This diet cuts most carbohydrates but allows for many fruits and vegetables, and later in the diet, actually allows some bread and other foods with moderate carbohydrate content. Unlike the Atkins Diet, it encourages lean protein and healthy fats. I did okay with this diet, and my cholesterol did not rise, but I struggled when the diet called for moderation. It allows for certain foods in

---

[3] Agatston M.D., Arthur. *The South Beach Diet: The Delicious, Doctor-Designed, Foolproof Plan for Fast and Healthy Weight Loss.* 2005.

prescribed amounts. I just could not always stop eating when I reached the allowed limits. I lost weight, though not as quickly as with the Atkins Diet, and I always gained it back.

In 2004, my wife, son, and I moved to Minnesota to be closer to family. I no longer have exact records, but I had already lost 20 pounds or more, at least 15 times. Over the next 5-10 years, I gained and lost weight several more times. I also started noticing the same pattern in my patients. (Far more common though was continued obesity and weight gain with no periods of weight loss.) Everyone can become frustrated with the food deprivations and hunger associated with weight loss, and rapid regaining of the weight typically follows.

Allina Health, the company I work for, started a program designed to improve fitness of the employees, including physicians. Since I already knew I was overweight, I figured that the program would not help me. In many studies, programs such as ours make little difference in the overall health of the participants. Our program included a fat percentage test. It is not perfectly accurate, but it told me what I already knew—I was fat. Seeing the number in print put to rest any of the stories we tell ourselves—we have more muscle than fat, we are big-boned, and so on. I decided enough is enough. My bad carbohydrate and junk food habit was like any other habit. To succeed, I had to give it up entirely.

Since that day, I vowed to give up junk food. But what does that mean? I realized I need a way of eating that is simple, that I can do forever. I want concrete guidelines of what I can eat, and which foods to eliminate. I realized carbohydrates were the problem, because starving myself is too difficult and studies show it also leads to muscle loss. But the Atkins Diet is too restrictive, and the South Beach Diet eliminates some carbs, allows for some foods in moderation, and becomes complicated. There are many other diet programs, but they have the same shortcomings. My own troubles and the daily interactions I have had with patients have taught me that simple, concrete rules are necessary. I came up with several rules that covered all of my requirements. Over time, I simplified and tweaked the rules, creating The Three Rules to Lose Weight and Keep It Off Forever.

I Know Why My Patients Do Not Succeed

As I was struggling with my own weight issues, the nation as a whole was getting heavier. Over the years, the average body mass index, a measure of a person's weight against their height, with 30.0 defining obesity and 25.0 defining overweight, has increased dramatically. My panel of patients reflects the national trends. I talked to my obese patients about weight at nearly every visit, but as a rule, they did not lose weight. I was surprised, but most just did not put forth the effort required. I think they did not realize how much work it takes to lose weight. There were a few who worked really hard and were able to lose weight, but like me, they usually gained it back, just as quickly as I did.

My recommendations to my patients mirrored what I was doing for my own weight problem. I started out recommending cutting calories, but no one liked going hungry, and no one liked giving up the high-calorie foods they enjoyed. Patients also usually lost muscle mass when they did manage to lose weight. As I learned the value of carbohydrate control, I started recommending it more and more, initially with the Atkins Diet. When patients diligently stuck to the Atkins Diet, they lost weight, but they usually quit before reaching their goal because the diet was too restrictive, and they quickly regained their weight when they went back to their previous habits. I still sometimes recommend the Atkins Diet, but only in the severely obese, so that they can lose some weight fast enough to feel a sense of accomplishment.

I then moved to the South Beach Diet and other similar diet plans, what some people call "modified Atkins Diets." I worked hard at convincing my patients, giving them my own summaries of the diets and recommending a few diet books. Some patients took my advice seriously and even bought the books. But they usually felt the plans were too complicated with too many things to remember. They had to learn lists and measure serving sizes, and they felt that they could not stick to the diet outside of their home.

I kept at it, knowing that carbohydrates were the key. (Later in this book, I will detail why the carbohydrate based plans work.) But people need a simple, inexpensive plan that they can follow without weighing and measuring food—a plan that allows them to eat at restaurants and with their friends and family. Over several years, I frequently tweaked my instructions, telling patients to ignore diets with multiple stages, to eliminate completely any foods that need to be measured, and to avoid expensive diet foods. I gave patients lists of foods to eat and foods to avoid, and I recommended more books to read. Slowly, more and more people lost weight. But still, most did not, and the majority who did lose weight gained it back. The diets were still too complicated and seemed too restrictive. Regardless of the method, losing weight is difficult.

A few years ago, I realized that I could eliminate nearly everything that my patients and I disliked about the carbohydrate-centered diets, everything that leads to failure and frustration and relapse. I made simple rules that when followed lead to success. I whittled the rules down to three, and I changed the wording about 20 times. I gave out summaries of the diet—just a few lines of text. I told them how to do it. I told patients that they could still eat and enjoy it, that they could still eat with friends, eat at restaurants, and eat inexpensively. I now teach everyone who will listen about my plan for eating—The Three Rules to Lose Weight and Keep It Off Forever.

This plan is still an effort, and most of my patients do not even start it. I understand why, and I don't really blame them. It is easier to just eat whatever we want, when we want. It is easier to make small efforts, but small efforts and half-measures do not work. You have to have very good reasons to work hard at something. If you put in the effort, The Three Rules work. Once in a while, a patient takes me up on it, applying The Three Rules to their lives. These people succeed. Today I saw a patient with diabetes. When I last saw him a few months ago, his sugars were okay, but not great, and he was taking two medications. I had told him about The Three Rules at earlier visits, and I went over it again. He took it to heart and started the plan. He came in today having lost 20 pounds—his weight is normal now, and he looks fit. His labs show completely normal sugars. It always surprises me when a patient puts in the effort, but when they do, it does not surprise me that The Rules Work. The complete resolution of his diabetes is not surprising either, since studies show that about 90% of diabetics who lose most or all of their excess weight go into remission, meaning that there is no sign of diabetes on the lab tests. Most go off medication completely, and I stopped one of this patient's medications today.

I have taught my son that you should almost never say never or always. So I will say only this: I believe that those who follow the Three Rules to Lose Weight and Keep It Off Forever will almost always be successful. It is possible that some people will follow The Three Rules closely and not lose weight, but I have not seen it yet. It almost never fails.

Introduction: What to Expect in this Book

Over thirty years of struggling with my weight, and nearly as long as seeing patients struggle, led to *The Three Rules for Losing Weight and Keeping It Off Forever.* In this book, you will learn how you can lose weight without hunger, significant deprivations, calorie-counting, measuring, counting carbohydrates, or medical intervention. Simply put, we avoid certain carbohydrates, what I call bad carbs. Soon, I will explain in more detail what carbohydrates are and which ones should be considered bad. For now, carbohydrates are sugars and molecules that we break down into sugars. You will easily learn what to avoid and what to eat so you can lose weight and not gain it back. You can do it right away, and you can do it forever.

This book is not for everyone. It is not for you if you expect an easy solution. You have to give up something. You cannot eat everything you like, everything you have eaten, that led to you becoming overweight, and yet still lose weight. The economist Thomas Sowell said, "Life does not ask us what we want. It presents us with options." You have the option of losing weight and keeping it off, *or* eating everything you want, as much as you want. If you choose the first option, then this book is for you. It will sometimes be difficult. But most people who have ever lived on this planet lived The Three Rules. They did it out of necessity. Still, if they did it, we can do it. For me, the benefits of weight loss followed by weight control are worth the effort. I hope it is the same for you.

I do not want to tell you The Three Rules and leave it at that. I want you to understand the problem of obesity, and why we should fight it. Do not be persuaded by those who say obesity is fine. Obesity is associated with a shorter life, worse quality of life, poor mental health, and a myriad of medical conditions. Yes, some obese people are content the way they are, but most would admit that they would rather lose weight, if they could. You need to know why it is so difficult to manage your weight. Before you adopt The Three Rules, you need to know about other potential solutions to the obesity problem and why these may or may not be for you. Since committing to The Rules is a big step, you need to first understand The Rules, why it works, and why it is the best option for most of us.[4] The Three Rules plan and this book are not perfect. As with any rules, there are gray areas. I have minimized them and have explained the few that remain. Do not get hung up on these very few minor issues. If you do, you will miss the larger picture.

Losing weight is always difficult, requiring serious effort and a change in many parts of your daily routine. I will go over some reasons it is so difficult. It will seem so hard that many of you will not want to put in the effort. Before you start, The Three Rules may even seem impossible. But most people, once into the diet for a few weeks, realize that while their routines have changed, it is not as hard as they thought.

The basis of The Three Rules is that certain carbohydrates cause nearly all of our weight gain. You do not want a science book, and I have not given you one. But you need to know how these carbohydrates cause weight gain, so you know why you should stop eating some of your favorite foods. I will discuss each Rule in enough detail so there can be no misunderstandings. The Rules work and they are simple, but there are a few points that will need explaining. Losing weight and keeping it off are different mentally, and you will learn how to do both. I do not want you to lose all the weight just to gain it back. It is demoralizing. There are pitfalls that can sabotage your plans and you will learn to avoid them.

---

[4] It is time to go over shortcuts and grammar. If I am talking about The Three Rules For Losing Weight and Keeping It Off Forever, I may refer to it as The Three Rules, The Rules, The Rules for Losing Weight, and so on. I will capitalize "Rules," so it is clear that I am referring to The Three Rules. I like to refer to The Three Rules as singular, because The Rules all go together, as one single plan, but sometimes it sounds wrong and I will use the plural. So usually, but not always, it will be "The Three Rules is…" Also, rather than say carbohydrate or carbohydrates over and over, I will usually write carb or carbs.

There are tips that help every minute and every day, while you are succeeding, and if or when you slip up.

Most importantly, you will know how to enjoy life under The Rules. You will improve your health, your quality of life, and your sense of well-being. As hard as it is to believe, you will love eating, maybe more than you do now.

Eating a certain way, to improve your health and accomplish your goals of weight loss and weight control, is just like accomplishing other goals in life. Over the years, I have succeeded and failed at many projects. I have been successful recently with my weight. I have been successful in my career as a physician. Mostly, I have been successful in my family life. But I have failed at many, many things: projects I have started and quit; a few friendships that have fallen by the wayside; family relationships that could be better. I have found that in these endeavors, it is discipline, focus, and planning that have led to the most success. Living by The Three Rules will help you lose weight and keep it off. But the concept of eating with intent and thinking about what you eat helps in all aspects of life—we succeed best if we think about what we are doing and do everything with intent.

I know that if you follow The Rules, you will lose weight. If you succeed, then I have accomplished my goal. If the concepts of The Rules help you with other parts of your life, then so much the better.

Part 1: The Problem

"It is the truth I seek, and the truth never harmed anyone."
Marcus Aurelius

People have gotten heavier. If you are my age, you remember that in school, there were a few obese kids and a few obese parents. You would hear people talking about how heavy a certain boy or girl or parent might be. Now, there are so many overweight and obese people, there is not much point mentioning a person's weight as a describing feature.

As I mentioned, the current definition of obesity for adults is having a body mass index or BMI (a formula based on the relationship of weight to height) of 30 or higher. Overweight is a BMI of 25 or higher. These are not new or more rigid definitions. The statistics are staggering. In a recent survey by the Centers for Disease Control (CDC) 42% of adults in the United States are obese[5], and over 70% are overweight or obese. Obesity is so common that what we see all the time, what we think of as "normal," is now overweight or obese. About 8% of Americans are severely obese, also called morbidly obese, defined as a BMI of 40 or higher. The statistics in children are equally alarming. Obesity in children is a BMI at or above the 95th percentile by standard growth charts. 18.5% of children and adolescents under 20, and 14% of children between 2 and 5 years old meet this definition.[6]

We will discuss some reasons for the increase in obesity, but first I want to go over the harms of obesity and why we should fight it. Some

---

[5] https://www.cdc.gov/obesity/data/adult.html
[6] https://www.cdc.gov/obesity/data/childhood.html

politicians and others talk about obesity's financial burden to society and the health care system. I don't care about that, at least not for the purpose of this book. I care about you and your health and well-being. You would benefit to know the potential harms of being overweight, so you can decide if the hard work needed to fight it is worth the effort.

There is a movement to accept obesity. I accept everyone. No one sets out to become obese. No one sets out to get cancer or any other illness. I accept and respect the obese and overweight, just like I accept and respect those with cancer and other illnesses. There are ad campaigns showing that obese people are beautiful. Of course there are beautiful obese people. There are beautiful people with cancer. But I still want to get rid of the cancer.

Negative Effects of Obesity and Why
We Should Fight It

If you do not understand the harms of something, why would you put in the effort to fight it?

It is a cliché that you have to want to quit something to succeed. That is true, but I don't think it is a helpful or sufficient sentiment. Many or most smokers in their hearts want to quit smoking, and many or most obese people want to lose weight. But that does not mean much. To quit smoking or lose weight, you need incentive enough to do it, so you can overcome the difficulties. I believe that the vast majority of smokers would quit in an instant if doing so would save the life of a loved one. Many would never smoke again if offered 10 million dollars. If offered the same threat or the same reward, most obese people would commit to losing weight, whatever the difficulties.

I am not at all saying that people with a weight problem don't want to lose weight. Just the opposite. I believe most do want to lose weight. If you did not want to lose weight, you would not have bought this book. But that is not the point. Do you have enough incentive to make the extreme effort that losing weight requires? It takes effort. But I don't think it is as extreme as it seems. Most people who lose the weight with The Three Rules in retrospect think it was not that hard. Looking forward, the effort may seem daunting. Looking back, not so much.

My goal in this chapter is to give you reasons to make the effort. Some facts are scary, but they are true. The truth does not harm us—the willful ignorance of the truth does.

Health Problems

Does obesity always lead to health problems? No, there are many healthy people who are obese. But that doesn't mean much. There are many healthy smokers, some living into old age. There are healthy people who drink too much alcohol, reckless drivers who have never been hurt, and drunk drivers who have never suffered the consequences. But it is undeniable that obesity increases the risks of many health problems. I expect that you already know most of these risks. Many health issues are especially linked to the pattern of obesity, with visceral or deep fat, the fat in the "apple" or "beer belly" pattern, being the worst, but just being heavy is a problem.

Type 2 diabetes (I will just say diabetes from here on), which used to be called adult-onset diabetes, is seen principally in the overweight and obese. By the time I graduated medical school in 1992, we did not see many adult diabetics. We did not consider this type of diabetes to be that big a deal, and we rarely needed to treat it with insulin. Now, in my practice, I follow over 200 patients with diabetes, and at least 90% are overweight or obese. There are genetic risks, but weight is the biggest factor. If you do not become overweight, diabetes is unlikely. If you have diabetes and you lose weight, the diabetes almost always improves, usually dramatically. As I mentioned in the previous chapter, improvement or remission of diabetes is the rule after weight loss. It is the most important thing.

Diabetes is associated with other health problems and is a leading cause of premature death. I have patients with diabetes who say that they are okay because they control their sugars with medications. But that only lowers the risk of certain diabetic complications—it does not eliminate it. It does not lower the risk of dying all that much. The best defense against diabetes is to lose weight and keep it off. Studies too many to count have shown the benefits of weight loss in diabetes prevention and treatment. It is the very first thing I mention to my diabetic patients.

If you are overweight or obese, and you do not have diabetes, you are not off the hook, not even close. Borderline or pre-diabetes, also linked to weight, is a serious problem. Many pre-diabetics have a condition called the metabolic syndrome. Blood glucose is mildly elevated, blood pressure is high, abdominal fat is increased, and the cholesterol is abnormal. Many people with the metabolic syndrome develop diabetes, but even those who do not are at significantly higher risk of heart disease and other problems.

Polycystic ovary disease is an increasingly common condition linked to obesity and diabetes. It can lead to infertility, excessive hair growth, and irregular periods. Weight loss and its benefits on sugar control usually help.

Fatty liver, also called non-alcoholic fatty liver disease, is often diagnosed in overweight and obese people and is uncommon in those with normal weight. Most physicians were unaware of this condition when I was in medical school. In fact, Eugene Schiff, MD, a renowned hepatologist, was my attending in medical school when we made the diagnosis of fatty liver in a non-drinker. It was such a novel disease that we presented it at a conference. Now, I see fatty liver every single day, often multiple times. While fatty liver often does not lead to any ill effects, it is so common in the United States that it is now a leading cause of cirrhosis, a serious, sometimes fatal disease.

Heart disease is far more likely in the obese. There are many obese people who have normal cholesterol and no heart disease, but remember that there are many risk factors, and obesity is just one. If you are obese, your risk of coronary disease and having a heart attack is higher. The strain that obesity places on the heart can also lead to heart failure, where the heart cannot keep up with demand. The legs swell and fluid builds up in the lungs. Patients have trouble breathing and abnormal heart rhythms often develop. Both coronary disease and heart failure can lead to sudden death. When you see a story about a celebrity dying suddenly, and the celebrity is obese, you are likely not all that surprised.

Blood clots occur more frequently in obese people. These can happen without warning or after major surgery. When the clots go into the lung, called a pulmonary embolism, it is sometimes fatal. When I hear of someone dying after surgery, especially if they were obese, I think of a blood clot.

Stroke, the devastating damage to the brain caused by a blood clot or bleed, is directly linked to weight, and reaching a BMI of 30 doubles the risk.[7] Losing weight lowers the risk. Strokes happen in thin people, but

---

[7] Kurth, T., Gaziano, et al (2002). Body Mass Index and the Risk of Stroke in Men. *Archives of Internal Medicine, 162*(22), 2557. https://doi.org/10.1001/archinte.162.22.2557

we see more and more obese stroke victims every year. Some people say that they don't mind dying, as long as they can eat the way they want. Well, stroke often leads to disability and complete dependence on others. I would give up some foods to lower that risk.

Atrial fibrillation, a common heart rhythm problem, can lead to stroke, heart failure, and other serious problems. The prevalence of atrial fibrillation is increasing, mostly because of obesity. In many impressive studies, weight loss markedly improves the success rate of treatment of atrial fibrillation.[8]

Sleep apnea, a serious and sometimes fatal condition where a person does not breathe effectively while sleeping, is closely linked to weight, and 90% of sufferers are obese. Sleep apnea causes daytime sleepiness, headaches, mental health issues, and high blood pressure. When I see an overweight patient who has these problems, I order a sleep study, first thing.

Arthritis, especially of the knees and hips, causes significant pain and disability, and is much more of a problem in the obese. It is well known and somewhat obvious that if someone puts more weight on damaged joints, it will hurt more, just as my knees hurt more when I carry a bag of water softener salt to the basement. It now seems that obesity can directly cause inflammation in multiple joints, even in the shoulders and hands. So obesity makes arthritis both more common and more painful. Anyone with arthritis understands the effect this has on their quality of life.

Worse outcomes in respiratory infections are linked to obesity. As I am proofreading this chapter, we are amid the Covid-19 pandemic. It has become clear that obesity is a major risk factor for severe complications and death from the Coronavirus. Over the next decade, when we look back at what we could have done to prevent some deaths from this infection, we may realize that being in better health would have been the best defense.

---

[8] Pathak, R. K., et al (2015). Long-Term Effect of Goal-Directed Weight Management in an Atrial Fibrillation Cohort. *Journal of the American College of Cardiology, 65*(20), 2159–2169. https://doi.org/10.1016/j.jacc.2015.03.002

You probably already knew about some medical problems described above, but this may surprise you—it surprises most of my patients. Obesity can lead to cancer. Some estimate that excessive weight causes 40% of all cancers.[9] It is not immediately intuitive, but obesity leads to cancer through inflammation and hormonal changes. Some cancers are much more of a risk than others, and for four cancers, obesity is more of a risk factor than smoking. As the rate of smoking falls, obesity may soon overtake tobacco use as the leading preventable risk factor for cancer.

I could go on for many more pages about the health risks of obesity—weight is linked to skin changes, fractures, asthma, neurologic conditions and many more. But some other consequences of obesity may be even more significant, and I will move on to these.

Quality Of Life

Just like the physical problems associated with obesity, the non-physical consequences do not affect everyone. Many, perhaps most people with weight issues are happy. But the fact remains that some overweight and obese people are unhappy because of their weight problem. Depression and anxiety are linked to weight, both as a cause and effect. Depressed and anxious people often eat more, and obesity can worsen or even cause depression and anxiety. This can lead to a cycle of guilt and depression, followed by weight gain, leading to more guilt and depression, and on and on. Even though there is a trend toward less fat-shaming, it still occurs. As she explains in her wonderful book, *The Willpower Instinct*, Kelly McGonigal details this problem in a way that hits home for many of us.[10] Overweight people may feel ashamed by what others think of them. The irony for many who overeat is that they cannot enjoy eating because of the guilt. I have heard many patients tell me they feel bad when they eat something that is fattening. They love ice cream, but even

---

[9] Steele, C. B., et al (2017). Vital Signs: Trends in Incidence of Cancers Associated with Overweight and Obesity — United States, 2005–2014. *MMWR. Morbidity and Mortality Weekly Report, 66*(39), 1052–1058.
https://doi.org/10.15585/mmwr.mm6639e1
[10] McGonigal, Kelly. (2012). *The Willpower Instinct: How self-control works, why it matters, and what you can do to get more of it.* New York, NY, US: Avery/Penguin Group USA.

in the privacy of their homes, they feel guilty about an indulgence. Again, this guilt can lead to even more eating.

Even without clinical depression, anxiety, or guilt, the quality of life of heavy people is affected. Many activities that young, fit people do are much more difficult for the overweight. My wife and I recently spent two weeks in Yellowstone and Grand Teton National Parks. We hiked miles every day and met many people on the trails. A few were overweight. A smaller number were obese. None were morbidly obese. Our national parks are wonderful vacations for so many people. Yet the best parts of these parks, the trails in the mountains, are virtually off-limits to those with a serious weight problem. The same holds true for other active vacations and activities. I don't see too many obese people on the bike trails or even the flat walking trails in Minnesota. The serenity of nature can be difficult to access for so many people. What do you do if you get invited by friends or family on a trip or activity that you know you cannot do? Unfortunately, this often leads to avoidance of these activities and loss of contact with others. It may seem impossible to imagine given the way your life is now, but when you get older and perhaps heavier, it is not at all unlikely. I see it all the time. I hope that if I am lucky enough to have grandchildren, I can go with them and our son on any vacation—of course, I have to be invited, which is another question entirely.

Maybe you are not interested or worried about the big trips. Maybe you don't care about hiking, biking, or even walking in the park. But since our physical strength worsens as we age, even activities that are simple now will become more difficult. Engaging with your family and friends can be a problem. You may not be able to play with your kids or grandkids. If you can do it now, can you imagine doing so when you are older and heavier? Will you be able to play catch with a grandchild? Sled with your nieces (if you are lucky enough to live in Minnesota)? Get in and out of the boat to teach your grandchild to fish? Work in the garden? So many activities will become difficult or impossible. So many people cannot engage in the activities that connect us to our families. So many people are missing out on life.

I have patients who because of their weight cannot easily live on their own. Even simple things like getting out of a chair, shopping in the grocery store, climbing stairs at a ballgame—they are all more difficult. Just watch people. The heavier a person is, usually the slower and more labored their actions. I have patients who cannot take their own shoes off to show me a foot problem. I help them put on their socks. These are examples that will not apply to many or most of the obese. But you get the idea. There are significant difficulties in being heavy.

But we can fight it. You have to want to fight it. You will need to find the reasons to lose the weight. Today is the best day to do anything important. Benjamin Franklin said, "Don't put off to tomorrow what you can do today." Start today.

Self-Image

Happy people usually have a good overall image of themselves. They believe that they are nice and pleasant to be with. They typically feel good about their physical appearance. I want that for myself and for everyone. But do happy people have a good self-image because they are happy? Or are they happy because they have a good self-image? Probably, it is a bit of both.

Despite all the media reports and celebrities telling us that fat is beautiful, many overweight people do not believe it. They may try to believe that they look good, but when they look in the mirror, they are not pleased. Again, this is not a rule. It may not even be true for most people, but it is true for some. I only mention body self-image to give you one more incentive to fight obesity and make the serious effort to lose weight. Self-image should probably not be the only reason for you to lose weight, but if it helps you, all the better.

If you do not have important reasons to lose weight, you will not make the effort, and you will fail. Everyone who loses weight feels better physically. Everyone who loses weight feels better about themselves.

Why Do People Become Obese?

Only humans, our pets, and our domesticated animals are obese. All other animals fight for their lives to get enough food.

In the distant past, to survive we had to eat what we could get. Like other animals in the wild, we ate nearly everything we came across that was not poisonous. Not that long ago, it was said that we had to work to feed our families. Now, far from starving, even the poor are often obese. That is a testament to the overall wealth of the United States and most of the developed world. With a modest salary, the price of food is not much of a factor in our caloric intake. We have plentiful high-energy food, providing us much more than we need. Yet we still eat as if we will never find food again. We do not worry about our next meal, but we keep eating. I call that eating without intent. We do not consciously think about what we eat. When we buy things without intent, we go into debt. When we eat without intent, we become obese.

On the other side of the energy equation, we use much less. Think about how much physical effort it took a hundred years ago to manage your home and your life. It is no wonder that now it takes genuine effort to avoid gaining weight. That would have been a laughable statement when our grandparents were born.

Often in the clinic, someone who has gained weight asks me to test them for a slow metabolism or a thyroid problem. They tell me they are eating the same as they used to eat and have gained weight. But if you are not measuring food, counting the times you eat out, and counting all the calories you burn, you don't know that you are doing everything the same. Some patients say that they eat what their friends eat, but they gain more weight than their friends do. But you don't see what your friends do when you are not with them. You may go out to dinner more than they do. You may get the large fries and they get the small. They may skip meals once in a while, or they may exercise more.

If it is so easy to gain weight, why are there any thin people? Most thin people today have had to work at it. They rarely eat junk food or they go on frequent diets. We think they are not fighting obesity, but we do not always notice what they do to stay fit. We may see them eat junk food once in a while. But for them it is a treat, and for us it is a habit. They eat at restaurants and eat junk food with us but eat differently when we do not see them. We may eat junk food at home, but they do not. Most of these fit people also exercise—a lot.

There are a few perpetually thin people who do not work at it. These people never eat too much junk food and never have second helpings. They never have the urges to eat the things that cause weight gain. I believe that these people just have a smaller appetite that is inborn or learned at a young age. Some do not crave sweets like other people. We are different, and they have an advantage over us in this aspect of their lives. Perhaps they have disadvantages, like motion sickness, migraines, or the cravings for something else, like alcohol. We cannot worry about people that are perpetually thin. We cannot worry about the reasons they are the way they are. We have our problems and they have theirs.

Most people have trouble maintaining a healthy weight in the modern world. We see it all around us. I want you to understand the reasons for this and how we can fight it. It is an effort, but you can do it. We cannot continue to do what we are doing and expect everything in our lives to change for the better. The world will not change for us.

Carbohydrates Are The Most Important

In nature, all animals struggle to get enough food. Most of the time, animals use energy as soon as they eat it. When food is more plentiful, the energy is stored as fat for later needs. Since food is scarce, animals in the wild rarely get so much food that they can store more fat than they will eventually need, so they do not become obese. People, until recently were no exception, and only a century ago, starvation was not uncommon, even in the United States. Like other animals, we developed a robust system for holding on to almost all the energy we eat, burning as little energy as possible, eating as much as possible, because days might go by when we would not have sufficient food to eat. Now, we have much more food than we need. We don't go days without eating, and many of us don't go hours. Our portions are larger, we eat more often, and the foods we eat are much more calorie-dense. A single bottle of cola has the calories of three apples. A medium coffee blended drink (basically a milk shake) has the calories of five apples.

What has changed the most in our diet over the last few hundred years is our carbohydrate consumption. Our total food intake has increased, but not at the same rate as carbohydrates, especially sugar and refined carbs like bread and bread-based products. Carbohydrates are the principal reason behind our obesity problem.

There are three categories of food: carbohydrates, fat, and protein. Carbohydrates are sugars and larger, complex molecules, such as starch, that our bodies convert to sugar. Sugars include **glucose,** which our body uses directly for energy; sucrose or table sugar; fructose from fruit; and lactose, in milk and dairy products. The various sugars have different effects on our metabolism. Multiple sources report that the average American eats 100-150 pounds of sugar a year, mostly in soft drinks, desserts, and other processed and prepared foods. In 1700, sugar intake was about five pounds per year. Our intake of starches has also increased, though not to the same extent as sugar.

Fats are found in plants and animals, acting mostly as storage for long-term energy use. Plant fats, except for coconut and palm oils, are liquids and include olive oil, peanut oil and the others. Most animal fats are solid at room temperature. We all have seen the fat on steak and bacon. Fats are high in calories, containing nine calories for every gram, while protein and carbohydrates have four calories per gram.

Protein is important in our diets, with animals being the largest source. Meat is mostly protein, with varying amount of fat and minimal if any carbohydrate. You can eat significant protein from plants, principally from the seeds. Plants also provide us with carbohydrates and fats.

Carbohydrates are the key to the obesity problem. Some carbohydrates, especially sugar, make fat storage easier, more efficient. Nowadays, too much of our diet consists of carbohydrates, especially the types that most contribute to obesity. Over time, nature favored humans who could gain weight easier, so we began to enjoy sugar and carbs, much like addictive substances. I have never had a problem with addiction to chicken, fish, steak or other meats and have never been hooked on olive oil. But I have had these issues with snack foods, bread, candy, pastries, and other high carb foods. We eat a lot of carbs because we like them, and we cannot stop once we start.

When we eat and digest food, the glucose level in our blood rises. Through multiple complex processes, we use the glucose and other compounds and store extra energy for later in the form of glycogen, a complex carbohydrate, and as fat. The higher the glucose rises, the more efficient the storage of fat. Since we are always using energy, if we are not storing fat efficiently, or at all, then we will burn it. So, even without exercise, we will often be in negative energy balance, meaning we burn more fat than we make. When we eat a lot of carbs, that doesn't happen, and it is more difficult to burn fat and easier to put it on.

We can survive without carbohydrates. We can make our own glucose from protein (and a little from fat) in our diet, and we can also use the energy we release from our own stores. There are historical peoples and even some in the world today who eat virtually no carbohydrate. Diets such as the ketogenic diet allow so little carbohydrate that our body enters ketosis, a process seen in starvation. In this state, we make ketones, compounds that our brain can use for energy instead of glucose. The ketogenic diet was around long before the obesity problem took off, being used in children for refractory seizures among other problems. People on these restrictive diets don't waste away to nothing, but they do not become overweight.

As you will see later, the very low-carb diets cause weight loss, even though you can eat virtually as much protein and fat as you want. Ironically, what we have historically thought of as fattening, say a cheeseburger, is fattening more from the carbohydrates in the bread than the meat and cheese in the burger. Peanut butter and jelly sandwiches are fattening because of the bread and jelly, not the high-calorie, high-fat peanut butter.

Because carbohydrates make fat storage easier, managing our carbohydrate consumption is the key to losing weight and the basis of The Three Rules to Lose Weight. Can you eat some carbohydrates on The

Three Rules? Absolutely. I eat almost all varieties of fruit, most vegetables, nuts, peanuts, beans, and most whole grains.[11] And I eat a lot of it—at least a cup of nuts a day, 2-3 pieces of fruit, lots of cheese and yogurt, and a vast amount of vegetables. My pressure cooker gets a workout with all the beans we eat. And remember, since protein and fat matter little to weight gain (if and only if you obey the Three Rules), I eat them every day. That includes all kinds of meat, chicken and fish, cheese, oils, and eggs.

So why does The Rules plan allow some carbohydrates but not others? Not all carbs raise our blood glucose in the same manner. Since the glucose rise varies by the type of carbohydrate eaten, the efficiency of fat storage also varies. The Three Rules allows you to eat the carbohydrates that do not cause a dramatic rise in glucose. What makes The Rules different from other diets is that you do not need to memorize lists of carbohydrates that you can eat.

There is a medical term that tells you how much our glucose level rises after eating—the **glycemic index**. Briefly, if you eat a food sample containing 50 grams of carbohydrate, your glucose will rise a predictable amount.[12] If you ate pure glucose, that rise is defined as 100, the highest you can get. Pure proteins and fats don't have any carbohydrate, and you could never reach the 50 gram amount, so you can forget it. They just don't raise blood sugar much, if at all. Each food can be tested, though not all have been. But so many have been tested that generalizations are possible. You may read that certain combinations of food result in a different glycemic index than eating them individually, but that effect is small enough that we can ignore it. The foods with a higher glycemic index cause more problems with weight than those with a lower index.

An additional point worth mentioning is serving size. We all know that candy bars are probably not good to eat if you want to lose weight. (That is more from the sugar than the fat or the calories.) But what if you had one small square of a candy bar rather than the entire bar? That

---

[11] We will talk a lot more about grains, since they have variable effects. Refined grains and all rice are against The Rules. There is more to follow, so don't worry about it now.

[12] https://www.gisymbol.com/how-is-gi-measured/

would be better. But as I will talk about later in the book, most people cannot stick to one small square. Remember that glycemic index is a reflection of a fixed 50 gram amount of carbohydrate. The term **glycemic load** takes into account the serving size. I do not belabor this point, though many diet books do. Some foods, like carrots, have a high glycemic index. But, there is so little total carbohydrate content in a carrot, you would have to eat a lot of carrots to reach that 50 gram amount. So carrots are fine. No one eats so many carrots at one time that it makes a difference.

Conversely, spaghetti is relatively low on the glycemic index, but typical dry spaghetti in the box has almost that whole 50 grams in one serving. And the serving size is 2 ounces, one-eighth of a box. When I used to eat spaghetti, I would split a box at most three ways. That is over 2.5 servings each. It is inconceivable to me to have a spaghetti dinner with one-eighth box of spaghetti. Fortunately, The Three Rules doesn't worry too much about serving size, as long as you are not ridiculous, doing something like eating 2 pounds of carrots at a time.

What about sugar itself? Sugar is probably the worst thing to eat if you want to lose weight and keep it off. In nature, there is not much sugar to be eaten. Fruits and vegetables have some, but unless you eat a ton of fruit, there just is not enough sugar to make people obese. Honey is basically liquid sugar, in its natural form, but there are few people in the world gorging on it. Honey is not allowed in The Three Rules, but I doubt anyone got fat on honey.

In the modern world, sugar added to food is the biggest problem. Foods with significant added sugar have a high glycemic index and glycemic load, leading to efficient fat production. In his superb book, *The Case Against Sugar*[13], Gary Taubes compellingly presents the argument that sugar is the root cause of obesity and many other serious medical problems we face in the United States, including diabetes, heart disease and even some cancers. If you want a reference for the history of sugar and the food industry and the dangers of eating food with added sugar,

---

[13] Taubes, Gary. *The Case Against Sugar*. First edition. New York: Alfred A. Knopf, 2016.

this is the best I have seen. The Three Rules eliminates added sugar and the other problem carbohydrates in a plan that is simple to follow.

We Don't Make Our Own Food

I am about fifty years old. When I was a kid, we did not eat out much. We made something quick for breakfast, and we usually packed lunch. We did not have snack-time at school, though sometimes we ate an apple. There was no takeout, and rarely did we eat packaged meals or pre-made meals from the grocery store. Think about your typical week and what the kids eat at school. How many meals do you eat at a restaurant, or from takeout or delivery? How many store-bought snacks do you eat? When you go to the gas station, do you get food? When I was young, there was only gas at a gas station.

It is estimated that on average one-third of people in the United States eat fast food on a given day. Some eat less than that and some eat more, but that is a lot. And many restaurants and takeout, which do not count toward that statistic, are worse than fast food. Several Panera Bread sandwiches have more calories and carbs than a Big Mac.

Why does this matter? The calories and carbohydrates are double or even triple in a restaurant compared to a home-cooked meal. Restaurants want everything to taste better than what you can make at home, so they add butter, sugar, (and salt) at higher levels than you would. The portions are bigger because they want you to think you are getting a good deal. Understandably they don't care about your diet plan or your goals.

I hear several days a week that eating at home is more expensive than eating out. That is not true. My wife and I will often share a half-chicken. Two chickens at Costco is about 10 dollars. That is five dollars a chicken, or $2.50 a half-chicken. I eat half of that for dinner—$1.25. If I eat a half-pound of roasted brussels sprouts or green beans (a large serving for either) that is at most another $1.50. Frozen vegetables are even less expensive at Costco. So my meal is under $3.00. Very few restaurants will cost you less than that. I don't even want to mention how cheap our soup night is. People say eating out is more convenient. Again, I don't believe it. I can make that chicken and vegetable dinner with a few minutes of preparation and then oven time. I can read, watch the news, talk to my wife or son, and so on. I don't have to drive to the restaurant, wait to order, wait for the food, wait for the check, and drive home. I enjoy eating out and I do eat out, but I don't do it to be healthier, to spend less money, or to save time.

You can lose weight with The Rules and still eat at restaurants. But you have to be more careful. Restaurant chefs only care that your food tastes good and fills you up. It can be high in sugar, other carbs and salt, though salt is not important for weight control. You may not know exactly what is in the food you get. They may not even tell you the truth of what is in the food. Controlling your diet is definitely easier at home.

Making more meals yourself will help you follow the Rules, save you money, and save you time. It is easier to have important conversations at home. You can be yourselves at home more easily than at a busy restaurant. I consider preparing meals and eating at home with my family an important part of my life, adding immensely to our happiness. I strongly recommend it.

We Get Little Exercise

I ask most of my patients if they get any exercise. Thankfully, some do exercise regularly, but a majority tell me that while they do not do formal exercise, they are active all day. I do not know what that means. They tell me they are up and down all the time, cleaning, mowing the lawn, and so on. None of those activities is what I mean by exercise. Mowing the lawn or playing golf burns more calories and does more good for your health than sitting on the couch eating bonbons, as my mother used to say. But compare this description of being active to what everyone did only 50 or 100 years ago.

People 100 years ago burned far more calories. We live a life of luxury by comparison. Most homes in the United States have dishwashers, washing machines, dryers, vacuum cleaners, electric irons, and on and on. Doing the laundry used to be a full day, grueling chore—chopping wood, feeding the wood stove, heating the water, scrubbing the clothes, putting the clothes on the clothesline, folding the clothes, and probably other steps I don't even know about. Not that I iron my clothes now, but if you have never picked up an old iron, they were very heavy. You had to heat the iron repeatedly over the stove and slide the iron carefully on the clothes until the iron cooled. Then you took a second iron off the stove and replaced it with the cool iron. It was laborious and burned a lot of calories. What we take for granted today as a minor task, was difficult work back then. It is easy to understand why most people were lean. You could not easily become obese with their diet and that level of exertion. If you ever became short on food, you lost weight.

In the past, usually only the wealthy would ever become over-weight—regular people were thin. Poor people starved. Only the wealthy had enough food to gain weight in significant amounts. Poor people to-day are not thin or wasting away, at least not in the United States or other developed countries. In fact, the poor are more overweight than the wealthy. Even poor people have electric or gas heating, laundry machines or access to a laundromat, and other modern tools to maintain the home. We have cars or public transportation, seldom walking any significant distance anywhere. In the past, the wealthy were sometimes overweight; they could afford rich foods and had thin servants to do the work and drive them places in their horse-drawn carriages. Now, daily work re-quires much less energy and all of us have access to energy-saving tools that did not exist 100 years ago.

Exercise is not one of the Three Rules to Lose Weight, but it is im-portant. Exercise burns calories and therefore fat. It is good for the heart, helps with stress relief, lowers the risk of multiple medical problems, and gives us a sense of accomplishment. Exercise helps us make the right food choices. I would feel foolish spending an hour on the treadmill and then having a bowl of ice cream. You do not need to exercise to lose weight, but it helps. There is no downside to exercise.

We Have Some Bad Habits

I think of a habit as something we do without thinking about it. Some of these are harmless, like cracking knuckles, humming to ourselves, and checking our smartphones, while other habits are serious and life-threat-ening, like smoking and drinking. I want to concentrate on the habits that are ingrained in our lives, are not that hard to break, and are unhealthy, but only in the long-term.

For any individual person, these habits may be easy or difficult to change, and may not even matter much to their overall weight or health. The main issue with many of our habits is the mind-set that they create. We have habits that reflect our thoughts on health and eating. If a person has a habit of taking the elevator one flight to their office and parking at the nearest spot to the front door, they may also be more likely to eat the muffin at Starbucks every morning, rather than eating an apple at home.

Many of our eating habits can be changed by just paying attention, doing things with intent. They do not require psychologists or medical intervention to break. Stopping at the coffee shop on the way to work is not subconscious or addictive, but I doubt many people really think it through. It is obvious that eating a scone or muffin every morning is worse for our weight than eating a piece of fruit, and that a caffè mocha has more calories than coffee and milk. But we don't think about it and keep doing it. Most people probably think little about the time and money spent every morning that they stop for coffee. I would expect that this habit could be broken if people added up the $4 and 15 minutes a day that we spend several days a week.

Similar habits are stopping at a vending machine on the way to your car, buying food at a gas station on the way home from work, grabbing samples at Costco, going to the snack drawer when you get home from work, and having dessert with dinner. We don't think about all the snacks we put out to watch a football game or the candy and cookies that are everywhere during the holidays. We do not think about the ice cream we have as a treat nearly every night. A daily treat is just a habit, one that can be broken by simply becoming aware of it. That is acting with intent.

Being active and exercising is a habit we can start just as easily. The concept of exercise and being active has changed dramatically over the last 100 years. Unless they live in a big city, people do not walk places. When I walk with friends to a restaurant or event, the limit for how far we will walk has shrunk. We automatically drive if it is further than a few blocks. The mindset used to be to walk, but now it is to drive. This is not a subconscious decision, but we certainly do not think it through. A mile walk to lunch gives you exercise, allows you time to talk with a friend, relaxes you, avoids the need for finding or paying for parking, and gives you a sense of accomplishment. If we do something without thinking about it, I consider it a habit. The first step to changing the habit is to decide if it is something you want to change.

Taking the elevator instead of stairs is another one. I know this habit is prevalent because it is uncommon for me to meet anyone in the stairwell of any building. If you think it through, the only negative of taking the stairs is the effort. Taking the stairs is quieter, usually faster because you don't have to wait for the elevator, and invigorating, especially in the morning. Again, it gives you a sense of accomplishment, and when we feel good about ourselves, we are more likely to do other things good for us, such as eating better. My colleagues mock me for my phobia of germs, but taking the stairs rather than the elevator avoids exposure to germs, especially important during flu season (and now, the Covid-19 pandemic). People and websites will tell you that you don't burn many calories taking the stairs. That is like saying there are few calories in a peanut M and M. Calories and energy add up for better and for worse. But that also ignores the other benefits. I want to develop healthy habits, regardless of the relative contribution of any individual habit.

There are many habits, such as drinking alcohol, that may require outside help to manage. The habits above are not that type. Doing more activities with intent, with knowledge of the benefit and harm, is very helpful. Think it through. Are there negative consequences to buying snacks, stopping for coffee and a donut, or taking the elevator? Is this a habit I can change? Just a few minutes of thought often leads to deep realizations.

It Is Hard To Lose Weight

If wishes were fishes, we would all cast nets.
Frank Herbert, in Dune

It makes sense that if it is so easy to gain weight, it is even more difficult to lose weight. Ads bombard us on television and the internet about effortless ways to lose weight. They are wrong. There are no simple ways. None. It is rare to achieve any important goal in life by an easy route. Weight loss is no exception. Either accept that it is hard, or fail in your attempts. I believe that The Three Rules is the best way to lose weight for most people. Like all methods, it is hard, but I think it is easier in the long run than the other methods. I have tried and have had some success with many methods of losing weight. They are all difficult, and generally, they all can be effective. Everything we do is a balance between the benefits and the downsides. I believe that all things considered, as hard as The Three Rules can be for some people, the benefits outweigh these difficulties.

Our Bodies Want To Hold On To Fat

For the same reasons we gain weight, it is difficult to lose weight. Our bodies are a product of millions of years of evolution. The world has been harsh on all beings, including humans, until recently. We struggled to get enough food, and when we ate enough, we stored it immediately, mostly as fat, so we could use it later.

Just like animals that hibernate, we store fat for the times when we do not have enough food. Since lack of food was common in the past, the easy storage of fat helped us immensely. We might go days without nourishment, certainly many hours, something not very common nowadays. That leaves us with extra fat and no lean times to burn it. Since we don't exercise as much as we used to, and we eat more than we used to, we have a lot of extra fat.

What happens when we starve ourselves, because we are stranded on a desert island, or we cut back intentionally? The same forces for survival want us to keep the fat as long as possible, because the starvation could last awhile. We need the energy, so we burn some fat and we lose weight. At least initially, most of the weight loss is fat. Later, we also break down some muscle, one downside of starvation diets. Soon, our body adjusts to the cut in calories, slowing our metabolism. That makes the total weight lost less than what would have been predicted. When we eat again at regular quantities, that slow metabolism allows us to gain weight quickly, a helpful trick in the past, when food was scarce—not so good now when food is everywhere.

Our body fights weight loss, and so do our minds. Evolution gave us a tremendous appetite. We were designed to eat *more* than we need for immediate energy use. It is as if we knew that we would have periods with inadequate food. We can eat, and often we do eat, whenever there is food around. Thousands of years ago, we could not afford to say, "I don't need to eat that apple or fig or leg of deer, I will eat something later." There may have been no food later. We could say that now, but our brain still thinks we shouldn't, so we feel hungry. This is the same reason that your pet Schnoodle will never turn down a treat. Hunger kicks in early in the dieting process, at least in most diets, long before you lose weight. You have to fight hunger for a long time, just to even start losing weight. Since your body adjusts to the lower intake of food, you continue to be hungry through the entire dieting process. It is difficult to fight a primal urge like hunger. When I used to lose weight by cutting calories, I knew that if I did not wake up hungry, the scale was unlikely to show weight loss.

Our bodies, through various metabolic mechanisms, want us to hold on to all of our fat. Our appetite wants to prevent starvation. And as we learned in the last chapter, the types of foods that are constantly around us make it easy to put fat right back on.

Times Have Changed

In the not too distant past, it was easier to lose weight. In fact, you had to work hard to get enough food to keep weight on. In the United

States and most of the modern world today, times have changed. As a percentage of our wages, food is much cheaper. Healthy food or junk food, it doesn't matter. You can get chicken for a couple dollars a pound. And you can often find two frozen pizzas for about 5 dollars on sale. If you make even 10 dollars an hour, you can easily feed your family for a day or two on an hour's wages. Since most of you reading this book make over 10 dollars an hour, you probably do not have to even consider the cost of the food you and your family eat.

Food is also much more available. If you live in a city, there is food at virtually every corner. It is nearly the same in the suburbs. On my six-mile drive to work, I travel one major street. There are over 20 food establishments and at least 10 of them are fast food. I am not counting five additional coffee houses. I am reading a Dickens book now set in the 1800s, and even the wealthy had just a few options for finding food in an entire small town.

At the grocery store, you used to buy groceries to make meals at home from scratch. Now you can buy all kinds of ready-made foods. The bakery section at the new monster store that went up near my house is bigger than the entire markets of old. Pre-made meals are so common that stores have a new name, "grocerants." Pre-made meals are usually more expensive than making it yourself, but they are still inexpensive compared to the cost of food in the past. Junk food is cheap.

The grocery store has healthy food—in the produce aisles, the "healthy" sections, and the meat and seafood areas. But the areas devoted to less healthy options have expanded. I love to grocery shop, so my wife seldom sees the inside of a store. She was recently surprised to see that the frozen potato section is an entire aisle. The other frozen vegetables fit in two freezers. There is far more ice cream than health food, by a wide margin. There is more candy than beans; more cookies than olive oil; more cereal than yogurt; more potato chips than hummus—you get the picture.

You do not need to buy the ice cream, prepared meals, pies, or candy, and no one is forcing you to eat it. But the more you see something, the more you will think it is normal and acceptable to eat it, and the more you will be tempted by it. I struggle to say no all the time, so I try not to get exposed to it. No wonder patients ask me "What do you eat?" when I tell them I don't eat what I call junk food. That is all they see when they shop. Using the alcohol analogy again—a recovering alcoholic should probably avoid bars and liquor stores, where every choice is alcohol.

Time is more of a factor today. We know that cooking at home is better for us, and likely less expensive. But with so many distractions and other activities today, it is difficult to manage our time. We know exercise is good for us, but we cannot find time for exercise either. Before smartphones, hundreds of television channels, streaming, and social media, we had less to do. Now, many of these distractions have become close to necessities. We think we have little time to cook or exercise, and sometimes we have less time, but we probably could carve out 45 minutes to prepare a simple meal and to exercise. It has become increasingly difficult to focus on these tasks with so much going on. Fortunately, The Rules require only a little time—a few minutes preparing simple meals, or a few seconds at a restaurant planning your dinner choices.

Our Minds Make It Harder

We all tell ourselves things that make it harder to lose weight. This may once have been a helpful instinct to get us to eat all the time, but it is not helpful now, when we are trying to lose weight. Our minds do the same thing with every habit, but when changing our diet, it may be worse, because food is everywhere. Again, a superb source for this aspect of losing weight is *The Willpower Instinct.*

Procrastination is the enemy of success in all things. In school, kids will do anything to avoid starting a project. The same is true for changing habits. Is there a good reason not to eat better right now? Why do we have to wait until tomorrow to avoid fast food? Is Thursday a better day to eat right? Or to exercise? Yet we all do it. We say that we will eat better tomorrow because today we are going out with Jane and John. Or I just don't have time to cook today. Or Teddy has baseball practice after school.

With my patients, I often use the analogy of alcohol or drug addiction. With a friend who is an alcoholic, would you advise them to quit alcohol tomorrow? "Tonight, drink up, tomorrow is an outstanding day to quit." It sounds silly. But we say that to ourselves with food. Tonight I will enjoy the burger and fries and I will start tomorrow. But tomorrow, there is something else to delay the start.

When we eventually start a plan to lose weight, our minds sabotage us. We make up reasons we need the cookie or the doughnut. We license ourselves to eat, when we know we should not. People in my office will run to get the free ice cream someone brought for Nurse's Week. We would not usually eat ice cream at 10 in the morning, but since it is Nurse's Week, then we do. Early January, patients blame their weight gain on treats at the office for the holidays. So a 50 cent cookie is okay to eat if it is free? If it were a rare event, that would not be a problem. But it is not a rare event. Treats can become almost a daily occurrence, and a daily treat is just a habit. In any diet, even The Three Rules, you must stick to it for it to work. We have all said to ourselves, "I know I shouldn't do it, but just this once." Then we know what usually happens next.

Our minds tell us it is okay to go off a diet because it is a holiday or a vacation. Why we should ruin our diet on a vacation, I don't understand. A recovering alcoholic knows not to drink alcohol on a vacation. And no one should cheat on their spouse because they are on vacation. So why would we cheat on our diet? But we do. A vacation is still our life. If it is important to do something, then it is important to do it on vacation. But our minds tell us otherwise.

We are also likely to go off our diet when we are upset, or something bad happens. Yes, getting in a fight with someone at work is upsetting. But it really has nothing to do with a burger and fries at McDonald's. Yet our minds make us think eating at McDonald's will decrease the anger we have at a colleague. The relationship between mood and eating is probably universal.

When a good thing happens, our minds also tell us it is okay to eat off our plan. We get a raise; it is okay to go out for chicken wings. Our boss praises us; it is ice cream all around. Logically, when something good happens at work, we should try to make ourselves even better. Yet our minds tell us otherwise, and we give ourselves the false reward of unhealthy eating.

Injuries can be even more mind-altering. I have never counted, but I would estimate that three times a week, a patient of mine tells me they have gained weight because of an injury. Perhaps they sprained an ankle five weeks ago. This somehow explains their six pound weight gain. Why they could not lift weights, do push-ups, slowly walk, or even bike, I cannot explain. Why an ankle sprain causes them to drink a Frappuccino or eat an ice cream sundae at Costco is also unexplained. But we all play these mind tricks, hurting only ourselves.

Logically, we know we should eat better starting today. We know we should exercise starting today. We know that a fight with a friend should not lead to unhealthy eating. Then why do we do what we do? Since eating and relaxing are so nice in the short term, our subconscious wants that pleasure to offset the pain or increase the pleasure of the situation. But we are logical, rational beings. To be successful in any diet plan, or any important endeavor, we have to overcome these natural urges. We can follow rules at all times, good or bad, on vacation or at work, in restaurants or at home.

With certain patients I bring up another difficulty of losing weight. I mention it here knowing that many of you will think I am wrong. Fine, feel free to ignore it and move on. In recent times, we have a different concept of hard work. So many of us, and I have sometimes been guilty, are unwilling to work as hard at something as is necessary. It is difficult to lose weight. Do it anyway. If a child tells a parent that the homework is hard, perhaps the proper response is, "Do it anyway." I dedicated this book in part to Ryan Holiday because his books, especially *The Obstacle Is The Way*, reminded me of this critical fact. Difficulty should not stop us. In fact, it should lead us to be better. Yes, it was hard for me to lose weight, each of the more than 20 times. It is hard to keep it off. With The Rules, I am doing it anyway.

Other People Make It Harder

It is clear you want to lose weight. Your friends and family would, if pressed, agree that you should lose weight. Yet the people around you often make it more difficult. Occasionally people secretly want you to remain overweight—perhaps to make themselves feel better. I think this malice is rare, and their interference in our weight loss is unintentional. Everyone has their own problems that they cannot solve easily. In part, when we see someone succeed, we feel a little insecure about ourselves, wondering why we cannot be successful. When our friend gets a new job, we feel happy for them, but it is tinged with envy. If a friend gets married, we might be a bit jealous. And when someone works hard and loses weight, that same envy can be there. Even without such thoughts, the people we know can make it difficult. They will not be on your diet plan, continuing to eat whatever they want.

You may have issues at home if you have a family or a roommate. You may have a goal of eating better, yet your spouse keeps chocolate chip cookies in the pantry. Your son comes home from college and absolutely needs to buy a box of Twinkies to roast at the fire-pit. (I am told they are better than s'mores.) Your roommate orders pizza, but you want something healthy. It is hard enough to eat right when it is just you. Like at a grocery store; if you are tempted enough times, you may cave in.

Work is even harder. Office colleagues bring treats. When you decline, they say, "One Christmas cookie won't kill you." One cookie won't kill you. But can you stop at one? Even one cookie could negate your diet successes of the day. These people do not mean to sabotage your diet, but that is what happens all too often. At the end of a day, you plan to go to the gym, but a friend asks you to go out for a drink. Even if you tell them about your exercise and weight loss plans, and even if they say they understand, you can see disappointment in their face. How often will you go with them instead of the gym?

When you have lost some weight, even a lot of weight, other things happen. Your friends may say how good you look and comment on your discipline, but with a subtle comment like, "I could never give up my bagel and cream cheese." Or, "don't you like beer?" These comments remind us of some things we have given up to accomplish our goals. I don't completely understand the psychology going on, but I think these people are justifying their own inability to give up certain foods or commit to a goal by pointing out what you are missing out on. I used to hear similar comments when I studied instead of partied in college.

If you want to succeed in weight loss or with any important goal, you have to understand the challenges and fight them. Say no to people offering treats—it will not offend them, and if it does, it tells you a lot about them. Tell your roommate you want to get something other than pizza; you may have to tell your son to keep Twinkies out of the house. Stick to your plans, regardless of the distractions.

It is Hard to Keep Weight Off

It is demoralizing to work for a year to lose weight, only to gain it back in a month or two.

In my struggles, I have gained as much weight as I have lost, except for the last time. The last time I lost weight, I stuck to the Rules and have kept it off since. In all, I believe I have lost about 550 pounds and have gained about 520 pounds. The weight loss took more than twice the time that it took for me to gain it back. Remember, our bodies want us to gain weight, to store energy for the times when there is inadequate food.

This is a brief chapter. We have already discussed why we become overweight and why it is hard to lose weight. The reasons it is hard to keep weight off are much the same. We gain weight back in the same way we gained it in the first place. But why do we gain it back so easily? Why is it so fast? And if we have put in all that effort to lose weight, why do we waste that struggle and just gain the weight back anyway?

Some reasons for gaining weight back so quickly are physical, such as metabolism changes, but most of the reasons are mental. It usually comes down to loss of focus on the problem. We do not pay attention to our diet at the same level that we did when we were trying to lose weight. We think we do not need to work as hard. In many ways, it takes more attention and more effort to keep weight off than it took to lose the weight.

We Don't Have a Plan

Most diets, such as the Atkins Diet and Weight Watchers, are designed just for weight loss. The diets may have maintenance programs, but they are not as intensive and are usually vague. I don't know too many people who are strict adherents to the maintenance stage of any regimented diet. Most people phase out of their diet, going back to their previous lives and habits.

About 10 times a day I discuss weight with patients. Some of them schedule their appointment to coincide with the start of a diet. This is especially common in January, with New Year's resolutions. They will talk about The Whole 30, the ketogenic diet, paleo diet, whatever. I encourage them, giving them a little guidance. But I always ask them what they plan to do after they lose the weight. Most of the time, they have given it little thought. At best, they say that they hope to make it a lifestyle change, rather than a diet (a common cliché, and effective, but rarely enacted). They hope to just stay on the maintenance phase of the diet forever, but it almost never works out that way. If they lose the weight, life gets in the way, and they do not stay on the maintenance plan. They may have had a plan, but when it comes time, it falls apart.

The key is to find a plan that works during the diet phase and after; a plan that you can stick to forever; a plan that can handle life and its inevitable challenges. You need a plan that is simple, so you can eat with intent, thinking about what you are doing at all times.

Our Bodies Adjust To Our Diet

Historically, we would lose weight by eating less, mainly when the supply of food was limited. Now, we only eat less if we are trying to watch our weight. Our bodies do not want us to lose weight because if we do, we may not have enough reserve to survive the times of inadequate food. If our weight is stable when we are eating 2000 calories a day, we will lose some weight when we cut our calorie intake down, say to 1500 calories a day. But, over the next couple months, our metabolism slows, and we burn less than 2000, maybe only 1600 calories a day. Our weight loss slows and sometimes we just give up. If we reach our goal for weight loss, we usually go back to eating the 2000 calories again (or more).

But now, we are no longer stable at 2000 calories per day. Since our bodies only need 1600 calories, we gain weight. Eventually that stops, as our metabolism reestablishes its 2000 calorie per day requirement. By then, we will have gained at least some of our hard lost weight back. If you eat over 2000 calories per day, you will gain even more.

Fortunately, The Three Rules and other carbohydrate-based plans have less of a problem in this regard. Weight loss can slow down, but not nearly as much as the low-calorie diets. The Rules are followed indefinitely, so even if your body adjusts and weight loss slows down, it really doesn't matter. You are unlikely ever to gain your weight back.

You may wonder why anyone would stick to The Rules diet plan when they don't stick to other diet plans. The Rules are different. The Rules are simple and easy to follow. You give up some foods, but there is so much you can eat, so much that you will enjoy, there is no reason to quit.

We Lose Focus

In anything, it is difficult to sustain focus long term. We throw ourselves into a project, paying attention to all the little details. After a while, we lose that intensity. We see this in sports, when a team wins in the beginning of the season, only to tail off in the home stretch. Students make careless errors at the end of a long exam. Dieting can be a lengthy process, but keeping the weight off is forever. You may watch everything you eat for a few months, even a year. Then you stop reading labels, you stop asking people what is in the food they are giving you, and you stop making healthy meals. A few bad days can lead to weight gain, at least a little. Then you can get discouraged and many people just give up. This is especially common in the diets that cause hunger. (Fortunately The Rules is not such a diet.) When you are hungry, it is easy to get distracted and eat whatever is near you.

A theme in this book and a helpful concept in life is to eat and do everything with intent. I keep that thought in my head most of the time. Do I skip a workout today? What will happen if I eat this cookie? Do I need it? If I don't work out, at least I thought about it, understanding the consequences of the decision. If I want to eat the cookie, despite the consequences, fine. I ate the cookie with intent. At least I am focusing on what I am doing. This is an excellent way to think about even minor day-to-day decisions. We usually take big decisions seriously, like marriage and changing jobs. I believe that we should do everything of any importance with intent, especially eating. We can prevent and change many unwanted habits by this simple technique. I tell patients that if you go off the Rules, do it on purpose, make it count. My choice would be cheesecake—nothing better. But I would do it on purpose, with a plan for what happens next. The rare time it happens, I immediately go back to the Rules. Much more commonly though, people lose focus, eat without intent, create a bad habit, and rapidly regain their weight.

We Think We Are Experts

People learn quickly, but we sometimes think we are better than we are. This happens at work, playing sports, investing in stocks, and in dieting. In any diet, including The Rules, you will lose weight, if you are strict, and it can soon seem to be very easy. In a low-carbohydrate diet, or a glycemic index based diet such as The South Beach Diet, the weight loss can be quick and dramatic. If you don't have a sizable amount of weight to lose, you can reach your goal in a few months or less. As I mentioned before, I have done this myself many, many times, only to gain the weight back.

When you reach your goal, you think you are an expert. How can the diet fail? How could I possibly gain it back? Don't forget that the millionaires in the stock market often think the same thing before the market crashes. Overconfidence leads to small changes in our habits. The stock investor makes increasingly risky trades, the young driver texts while driving, and the dieter thinks they can have one snack or meal off the plan. It starts with a large fries at McDonald's, one Thin Mint Girl Scout cookie, or my nemesis of the early 2000s, the Sourdough Jack Burger at Jack In The Box. (Don't eat one, you will be addicted.) You say to yourself that you know what you are doing, and you can have it just once. You can, for a while. But then you are doing it a few days a week, then every day. At one point, I had an iced latte and coffee cake at Starbucks every morning and a Sourdough Jack Burger most afternoons driving to pick up my son after work.

Every time I have ever gained my weight back, it was because of overconfidence. I thought I was an expert and could just make a few changes to my healthy diet. Weeks or months later, after gaining most or all of the weight back, I would admit to myself that I was no expert and would go back to a strictly enforced diet plan. I would lose weight, and the cycle would then repeat, often with the same temptation, the Sourdough Jack Burger.

We Think We Can Eat In Moderation

When we reach our goal with a diet, we rarely think that hard about how to keep it off. A common answer when I ask a patient what they plan to do, if they don't mention the rarely followed maintenance phase of a diet, is that they will "eat in moderation," or "eat sensibly." You have heard that many times. It works, if you can do it. But if you could eat in moderation all the time, you would have done it and would not be overweight. This is like the sage advice of an investment expert—buy low and sell high. Expert advice, except how do you know when the stock is low or high? With food, my idea of moderation may not be the same as yours. Similarly, I have had many patients tell me that moderate drinking is a six-pack of beer at night. I don't have that same definition.

With eating, I have seen advice for dieting to keep the calories under 2000 a day. That may work for some, but it can cause weight gain in others, depending on what you are eating to get the 2000 calories. In addition, if you are not measuring and weighing food, you are likely eating more than what you think. You might say that a moderate dinner is one serving of chicken breast and one serving of white rice. But if you don't measure it, your chicken breast may be one and 1/2 servings and your rice three servings.

Despite the arguments of old school dietitians, what you choose when you eat in moderation makes a difference. With the standard 2000 calorie a day recommendation, a 2000 calorie diet of lean meat and vegetables is a good day. A 2000 calorie diet of pastries and pasta is not. We store fat more efficiently with sugar and refined carbohydrates compared to meat and vegetables.

The biggest problem with the recommendation of eating in moderation is that even with the best intentions, it is difficult for most of us. Try to tell an alcoholic to drink alcohol in moderation. Can a drug addict do drugs in moderation? I cannot eat in moderation. One cookie leads to the next. My wife can eat one bite of cheesecake or just a few M and M's. It is annoying watching her do it, since I cannot do it myself, at least not reliably. How many times do we tell ourselves, "just one bite"? We know that a moderate snack would be a handful of nuts or a few chips, but we keep going back. I call that eating from the trough, and I will talk about how to avoid it in The Three Rules. I will give you a hint—it involves the analogy of alcohol again.

We Do Not Realize That Sugar and Carbohydrates Are Addictive

Anyone reading this book has had a weight problem or knows someone who does. I have it under control currently, but that has been far from the case for most of my life. Most of us will attest that it is hard to eat less sugar and refined carbohydrates. It is hard to have one Oreo cookie. Since we store fat efficiently when we eat sugar and carbohydrates, this is a genuine problem.

When I mention the low glycemic diets and The Three Rules, virtually all my patients do one of two things. They either say, "I love carbs." Or they think, "I love carbs." We developed a taste for carbohydrates over thousands or even millions of years. Lions like meat, we like carbohydrates. That is how our species has survived. With all the other wonderful traits of humans that have helped us—intelligence, opposable thumbs, and the love for our family—we also developed a love of sweets. This has helped us survive—until recently.

But are sugar and refined carbohydrates addictive? Some studies suggest they are, and experts are divided on the issue. I again point to Gary Taubes's superb book, *The Case Against Sugar*, if you want to read about sugar addiction. But I don't really care about the science in this instance. Whether sugar and carbs are as addictive as cocaine doesn't matter to me. Sugar acts like an addictive substance. There are many definitions of addiction, but I consider something addictive if we do it despite the negative consequences; we try to stop and have trouble; we hide our behavior from others; or we are embarrassed by the behavior. I knew many years ago that sugar and carbs were making me gain weight. I remember hiding candy wrappers from my parents. I have been embarrassed when I had to admit to my wife I had a large fries at McDonald's when I bought our son a Happy Meal. I know this is not the same as sneaking Johnny Walker at work, but it sounds like an addiction to me.

The point is not whether it is more difficult to quit sweets or drugs. But if you don't recognize that sugar and processed carbohydrates act like addictive substances, you will be tempted by a small treat. That is fine for some people, but not for most of us. We don't stop at one. That leads to a rapid increase in the consumption of these foods. Then, most of the hard work is ruined, and you gain your weight back, usually quickly. The All or None approach works for other addictions, like alcohol. It works for sugar and refined carbohydrates. In the past, I have eaten all—now I eat none.

Part 2: Possible Solutions

Every diet works, if you can stick to it. That is the rub.

I have already discussed some methods people use to lose weight. There are countless books, magazines, websites, and videos devoted to one diet or another. Every popular diet will cause weight loss, since if the diet did not work, it would not be popular for long. I have lost weight by most methods—cutting back, calorie counting, low-carbohydrate diets, and extreme exercise.

I lost weight faster in some diets than others, but they all worked when I stuck to them. That is the problem—all plans stop working if you stop following them. The key is finding a plan that you can stick to. You should learn about the various options. Some you can do on your own and some involve a physician, with supervised plans, medications, or surgery.

Most do-it-yourself plans are difficult to stick to, while physician managed plans are often restrictive and expensive and are not usually used long term, so regaining weight in both settings is typical. Medications for weight loss should not be taken forever, so again most people gain the weight back when they stop the medications. Weight loss surgery works and has reasonably good long-term data supporting it. But it is drastic, changes how you eat forever, and has substantial risks.

In this chapter, I will go over some of these methods for losing weight. They may be right for some people, and they may work for you. In my experience with my weight problems and with my patients, there are too many failures with these plans for me to recommend them widely. I want a plan that is safe, will work the first time, and work forever. The

Three Rules is hard, but it is such a plan. If you follow it, you will still enjoy eating, you will lose weight, and you will not gain it back. You will also have the satisfaction that you did it on your own. That will help you in other aspects of your life. If you can lose weight on your own, what can't you do?

Eat Less

My doctor told me to stop having intimate dinners for four.
Unless there were three other people.
Orson Welles

Historically, we dieted by eating less. Even before the word calorie was used, people knew that if you ate more, you would gain weight. If you ate less, you would lose weight or at least not gain. It is not the weight of food that matters but the calories, the amount of energy food has. A full plate of cabbage has fewer calories and less potential for weight gain, than a small plate of cheesecake. Before we started eating so much sugar and carbohydrate, calories eaten and burned explained most of weight gain and loss.

In general, eating less will cause people to lose weight. That is obvious. I have heard people, even health professionals, say that someone who is struggling at weight loss is not losing weight because they are not eating *enough*! That is not true. Think about it. When a person eats nothing, they waste away and starve to death. If you feed them, they stop losing weight and eventually gain the weight back. If zero food causes weight loss and starvation, how could it be that not eating enough would cause weight gain or interfere with weight loss?

Eating less definitely helps with weight loss, but trying to fight appetite, our biggest urge, usually fails. Eating less is the basis of the diets I will discuss in this chapter. These diets work for many people, though often just for a short time. You are welcome to try these diets—I have. If you want a plan that works, is easier than just eating less, and lasts forever, I would look elsewhere.

Just Cut Back

Can you cut back on what you eat and lose weight? The idea is simple. Eat less, by cutting portion size, minimizing snacks, or eliminating certain fattening foods. I had a friend who could just quit drinking alcohol for a few months and lose weight. When I ask patients if they are trying to do something about their weight, they often say that they are just cutting back on portion size. Sometimes, cutting back is effective, but usually it takes more effort than that. Often, a young, very active man cuts back and is successful. He stops eating desserts and second servings at meals. He may give up fast food or eating out entirely. The most successful will sometimes tell you that is all that they have done, and they may even believe it. But if you delve deeper, you usually find that they also gave up alcohol, sugary drinks, and refined carbohydrates. They may have even started working out nearly every day. A lifestyle change that involves cutting back, giving up carbs, and exercise works, but very few people do all that.

There are some fortunate people who can lose weight by cutting back on what they are eating and changing nothing else, except perhaps a little more exercise. I am very happy for them. The problem is that they usually cannot keep it up. They generally experience the yo-yo effect. They go on vacation and eat the sweets again. They get busy at work and stop exercising. Stressful life situations lead to drinking alcohol. And so on. Then they gain the weight back and have to start over.

Far more common is that you try cutting back, not realizing how hard it is. (See the earlier chapter on the difficulty in losing weight.) You hear of a friend's success in cutting back and you try it. You may not put in the effort that your friend did—maybe you still have wine, still don't exercise, and still eat out too much. You fail and feel bad about yourself. Sometimes we think there is something medically wrong with us, that our friend lost weight cutting back and we cannot. But often they were doing things that we are not doing, and in any case, not everyone is the same. Some people can do certain things better than other people, in weight loss and in everything else.

Losing weight is hard. Cutting back a little on what you eat is fairly easy, but it rarely works. When it does, it is not sustained, and you will probably gain the weight back quickly. If you are overeating, you should cut back, but don't expect a major improvement in your weight. There are better ways to lose weight in the long run.

Calorie Counting

What about formal calorie counting? You can have some success in counting and cutting calories. It seems simple—eat fewer calories than you burn. Some smartphone apps allow you to scan barcodes of products, search vast databases, and track calories, fat grams, carbohydrate content, and vitamins with no effort. Tracking calories is not the problem.

The first issue is how low does your calorie count need to be for you to lose weight? Everyone is different. I am about 5 foot 5 inches. 2000 calories a day might cause a man 6 foot 5 to lose weight, while I would gain weight. We also know that not all calories are the same. 1800 calories a day of protein, vegetables and some fat would cause weight loss. 1800 calories of mashed potatoes and pie would not. In addition, our energy expenditure affects the success of calorie counting. 100 years ago, when people burned thousands of calories a day managing their home, a person might lose weight at 2200 calories. Today, with the help we have doing every chore in the house, you would probably gain weight at that calorie intake. That all said, though, virtually everyone will lose weight if they consume less than 1200 calories a day.

Most people who plan to count calories eat more than they think. We talked of serving sizes earlier in this book. A serving of boneless, skinless chicken breast is less than one chicken breast. A serving of pasta is ⅛ of a box. If you are not measuring and weighing your food, you are likely underestimating what you are eating. With the analogy of alcohol, when I ask a patient how much they drink, when they say, "two drinks" and they are not measuring, they are usually drinking two rather large drinks, more than the standard 5 ounces of wine or 1.5 ounces of spirits. So when someone tells me they are not losing weight and they say they are eating 1100 calories a day, the first question I ask is whether they weigh and measure their food. If not, then I know that they are undercounting. People also don't realize that if you are counting calories, every calorie matters. The small sample at Costco, the coffee creamer in the morning, the few fries from your son's dinner—that all counts. 1200 calories is not a lot. A few uncounted bites, each at 40 calories, can make a difference.

Calorie counting is difficult enough, but being hungry is the hardest part. Remember from before, we have powerful appetites, and they have to kick in *before* we lose significant weight. If that were not the case, we might not eat until after we already started losing weight. That would lead to starvation, if the food we just decided not to eat happened to be the last food we would see for several days. I mentioned before that when I was calorie counting, I knew whether I had lost weight before I got on the scale in the morning. If I was hungry, I had lost weight. I dislike the idea of being hungry for weeks or months, while I am trying to work and enjoy my life. What if I want to eat out and I already had 900 calories? That leaves only a few hundred calories for dinner at a restaurant. A salad is about all there is, and that is with a low-calorie dressing—on the side.

Even if it works initially, the body adjusts to a low-calorie diet. If you are eating 1200 calories a day, your body adjusts nearly to that level, after only a few months. Now, eating much over 1200 calories might cause weight gain. I don't think you want to count every calorie you eat for the rest of your life just to avoid going over 1200. We usually start eating over 1200 calories, even back to our original 1800-2000 and gain weight back. This is detailed in earlier chapters, and this problem derails most calorie-cutting diets over time.

Weight Watchers

There are several commercial programs and systems to lose weight, involving various methods of cutting back on how much you eat. Some talk of portion size, others teach you to eat only when you are hungry, and others have you divide meals into different categories. You check in with their advisers, who help keep you on task. Weight Watchers, the most popular system, assigns points based mostly on calories. Some foods, mainly fruits, vegetables, and pure proteins, don't count at all.

Many of the programs, including Weight Watchers, meld a typical calorie-cutting diet with a low carbohydrate or low glycemic index diet. There is much to like about these systems, especially that they hold you accountable with frequent check-ins with advisers. But you still have to count points or otherwise pay close attention to what you are eating, and to do so accurately you have to weigh and measure. That is difficult at restaurants and becomes tiresome at home. You still have to eat in moderation, holding yourself to a small serving of something you like. A food choice may have 10 points, but only if you measure it correctly and do not have seconds or thirds. A system may say to only eat when you are hungry, but we already knew that. Again, if we could eat moderately, we would not need a diet at all.

The biggest problem is what you do if you reach your goal. What next? When I ask patients this question, they usually say that they will either continue on the maintenance program or just do the system on their own. Later, perhaps at the next yearly physical, most of those on Weight Watchers will have lost some weight, but not all they intended to lose. Most will have stopped the diet because of cost, time factors, or lack of interest. Over the next year or two, the majority will have gained their weight back. I have seen only a few patients have long-term success with Weight Watchers or similar plans.

Intermittent Fasting

I will briefly mention intermittent fasting. There are many forms of this diet, but they all work the same way. You pick times or days when you eat little to nothing. The other parts of the day or week you eat normally. For example, you may only eat during an 8-hour period each day, fasting the rest. Or you might eat very little two days a week and eat moderately the other five days. This 5/2 ratio is the basis of one of the most popular intermittent fasting diets. Over the course of a day or a week, you will cut enough calories to lose weight. You may also trigger some very healthy processes in the body. Studies confirm that many people lose weight this way, and there may be additional health benefits, unrelated to weight loss. For some, it is easy and enjoyable, but most people don't reach their goal, and few keep the weight off. I want to discuss the weight loss aspects of the diet. The health and other benefits are a separate issue and may very well be worth exploring for some of you.

In the actual world, things are different than in studies. People are often more strict with their diet when in a study, and just being willing to participate in such a study requires a level of commitment we do not always see outside of a study protocol. There are at least three problems with intermittent fasting as it applies to weight loss. First is that some people overeat during the periods they are not fasting. If you are on the two day/five day intermittent fast, you may overeat enough during the five days to balance out the two days where you eat little. You can become discouraged because you suffer during the fast and don't end up accomplishing much.

Another problem is that the fasting periods can be very difficult. Remember, if you could easily tolerate fasting and hunger, you likely would not be overweight in the first place. This has been my problem when I have tried intermittent fasting. I am hungry, and I don't function very well hungry.

In my mind, the biggest problem with this diet approach is social. What about travel? What if someone wants you to eat with them during a fast period, such as on vacation? What about long term? Do you want to be on such a regimen forever? My patients on an intermittent fast will often come back from vacation, not having followed the plan. They may have gained some weight back and hope to get right back into the intermittent fasting, but it doesn't happen. I have yet to have a patient stay on an intermittent fasting program long enough to lose all the weight they planned. If I have seen anyone lose weight and keep it off after one year, I do not recall it.

Jenny Craig, Nutrisystem And Others

I have tried Jenny Craig, Nutrisystem, and similar programs before, and lost weight every time. As most of you know from ads or from trying them yourself, you eat the food that they make. In some plans, you eat their food exclusively; in others, you supplement their food with healthy meals you make yourself. These plans are somewhat regimented, so you have little opportunity to stray from what they tell you to do, unless, of course, you eat food other than what they send you. When I tried such a diet, not being that picky, I did not have any problem with the taste or quality of the food. The meals and snacks are low-calorie, either because they are very healthy, or they are just small servings of less healthy food. So, like most diet plans, they work by making you eat less.

These plans are low-calorie diets, though some programs have low carbohydrate and low glycemic options. The major benefit is that they do nearly everything for you. You just follow what they tell you. There are sometimes coaches and mentors, and that helps. I already mentioned a flaw. It is still up to you not to stray from their plan. What if you want to go out to eat? What if you travel? What if you are hungry, despite eating all your meals and snacks for the day? If I have the willpower to eat only healthy foods in moderation, it is not the actual preparation of the food that is the problem. I can look up a recipe, calculate the right serving size and make it myself. My challenge has always been eating food, healthy or not, in moderation, regardless of who prepares it.

Just like Weight Watchers, you also have the problem of what you do when you are done. Even if you stick it out for several months, eating only their food, and you lose the weight you hope to lose—then what? Are you going to eat their food forever? Some quit the program and make the foods they remember eating for the past few months. If you are not careful, and you do not weigh and measure, you are likely to overeat. If you can make sensible meals and not stray, then why were you not successful when you have tried to do that in the past? These diets can be more difficult in the long run than Weight Watchers because even if you are successful, you have not learned how to lose weight and keep it off without the help of someone else making your meals. With The Three Rules you learn how to do it, and you learn right away. Follow the Rules and you will succeed. That is all you need to learn, forever.

Meal Replacement Diets

Jenny Craig, and other plans make meals for you to eat, hoping you won't also eat your own food. Meal replacement plans are more extreme. They give you food but not traditional meals—usually shakes, bars, and puddings. Years ago, at least twice, I lost weight on SlimFast. There are now a few different systems in SlimFast, and the shakes have changed, but the concept is that you drink their shakes, usually twice a day. When

I did it, you were told to make a sensible dinner. Like all diets, SlimFast and similar programs work, if you stick to them. The appeal of such a plan is that for most of the day, you don't have to think about what you eat. You drink their shakes, which I enjoyed, and forget about food. I could do it for a while, but then I would always slip up. I overate when I went out for my "sensible dinner," when I went on vacation, or after I got bored with the shakes.

Some such programs are more restrictive, and some have some medical supervision. You meet with nurses and doctors and use their meal-replacement products. Other than the supervision, which is supposedly tailored to your individual needs, there is not much difference between doctor-supervised meal replacement diets and the ones you do on your own. The cost of the supervised plans is more, and you cannot usually buy their products online or at Target, as you can with the other diet plans. They are low-calorie, usually less than 1000 per day, and the evidence shows that these diets work. But again, the long-term success rates are not very high, for the same reasons the do-it-yourself programs often fail. No one stays on them forever. I have nothing negative to say about supervised meal replacement programs in general. These programs are the same as almost all the others. Almost all diet plans work while you are doing them and fail when you go off of them.

If you eat less, you will lose weight. It doesn't matter if you count calories, join Weight Watchers or any of the other programs I mention. But the same problems arise in all of them. What have you learned from the diets? Do you want to be hungry forever, and are you going to drink two or three shakes a day forever? What about travel, restaurants, and the simple boredom of eating their food? Most people regain a significant proportion of their lost weight soon after stopping the diets, even if there is a maintenance program offered. The best way to lose weight and keep it off is to have a single plan that works forever. Sure, you have to stick to it, but The Three Rules will work as well or better than these diets, it is essentially free, and it never stops working. Sticking to Three Rules is much easier than buying shakes or special meals for the rest of your life.

Exercise

*Exercise will help you lose weight. But to overcome a poor diet,
it takes a lot of exercise.*

Exercise burns energy. As we know, if you take in more fuel (calories) than you burn, you will gain weight. We have discussed that certain foods may change how efficiently we gain weight, but the calorie concept is still generally true. So doesn't it make sense that burning more energy will help with weight loss? Yes, of course exercise helps with weight loss. But it is difficult to exercise enough to lose weight and keep it off. It can be done, and I know many people who have done it. But it takes hard work, consistently, forever.

Should You Exercise?

It has been known for generations that exercise is good for us. I cannot think of any medical condition harmed by exercise. Cardiovascular exercise, such as running or biking, and resistance training, such as weightlifting, both help prevent disease. Exercise can lower the risk of heart disease, stroke, cancer, depression, erectile dysfunction, low back pain, and on and on.[14] [15] A recent extensive study confirmed what we already knew, that moderate exercise saves lives.[16] I recommend exercise for nearly every patient.

The greatest benefits may be mental. We get a feeling of accomplishment from exercise, making us happier and more likely to do other

---

14 Esposito, K., et al (2004). Effect of Lifestyle Changes on Erectile Dysfunction in Obese Men. *JAMA*, 291(24), 2978. doi:10.1001/jama.291.24.2978

15 Thorogood, A., et al (2011). Isolated Aerobic Exercise and Weight Loss: A Systematic Review and Meta-Analysis of Randomized Controlled Trials. *The American Journal of Medicine*, 124(8), 747-755. doi:10.1016/j.amjmed.2011.02.037

16 Kraus, W. E., et al (2019). Physical Activity, All-Cause and Cardiovascular Mortality, and Cardiovascular Disease. *Medicine & Science in Sports & Exercise*, 51(6), 1270-1281. doi:10.1249/

healthy things for ourselves. Exercise also relieves stress and anxiety. If I am struggling to keep up with my wife when biking up a hill, or working to keep up with my son and nephew hiking in Montana, I am not worrying about other things in my life.

Nearly every healthy person benefits from exercise. When a patient sees me for an ailment, more often than not, I recommend exercise as part of their recovery. Since exercise is difficult, most people exercise much less than recommended. The concept that exercise is good for us has been known for quite a long time, and I doubt I need to convince you. But will you lose weight if you exercise and do not also change your diet?

Exercise And Weight Loss

Exercise helps people lose weight[17], but less than you probably think. In multiple studies, exercise alone results in a loss of about 3 pounds and an inch of waist circumference. I have seen over the years many people who have failed to lose significant weight or who have actually gained weight, despite fairly rigorous exercise. If you look at charts that show calories burned with exercise, or if you look at the displays on the exercise machines, you can burn a few hundred to 600 calories with an hour of exercise. I believe that the machines overestimate the calories burned, but even at face value, that is just not a lot of calories. If you work out 45 minutes and burn 300 calories, you can negate all of it with a Gatorade, a smoothie, or a single snack. We eat far more food than our body needs, and 300 calories burned just doesn't amount to enough energy to counteract our eating.

Remember that many years ago, the average person did far more than 45 minutes of exercise just getting work done around the house. And that was while eating fewer carbohydrates and much less sugar. With the modern diet and our leisurely lives, this level of exercise will not cause dramatic weight loss. Most people do little or no hard exercise routinely.

---

17 Thorogood, A., et al (2011). Isolated Aerobic Exercise and Weight Loss: A Systematic Review and Meta-Analysis of Randomized Controlled Trials. *The American Journal of Medicine*, 124(8), 747-755. doi:10.1016/j.amjmed.2011.02.037

Many of my patients say they walk 10000 steps as measured by a wrist monitor. 10000 steps during a regular day is not at all like an extra workout of 10000 steps of running or even power-walking. Before you started measuring, you may have been walking 6000 steps, so an additional 4000 steps walking around the office will not do much. If someone exercised two hours or ran 10 miles every day, yes, that would cause weight loss, but that is not reality for most of us.

I am not at all saying you should not exercise. Everyone should. The benefits are enormous, and I will go over them in more detail later in the book. I have never felt bad about myself after exercising. I have never regretted working out. But, I know that while exercise helps us lose weight and keep it off, it is nowhere near as important as what we eat.

Carbohydrate Based Diets

We all like sugar. That is a fact. It causes weight gain. That is another fact.

From what you have already read in this book, you know that I am against eating sugar, at least food with added sugar. There is no question that in the quantities we consume, it can lead to obesity, diabetes, and many other illnesses. Cutting added sugar and certain other carbs out of your diet helps. I have already mentioned the Atkins Diet and the similar ketogenic diet, the prototype very low carb diets. These diets work, and I have mentioned how they can fail in the long-term. I want to expand on these diets a bit, because they are very tempting. I will also go over the low glycemic index diets that arose from these very low carb diets. The Three Rules is based on the glycemic index, but as you will see in later chapters, it is simpler and avoids the pitfalls of the diets I describe here.

Very Low Carb Diets

Robert Atkins should be commended for popularizing the idea that cutting all sugar and nearly all carbs from the diet results in weight loss. The original Atkins Diet allowed for very little carbohydrate, often fewer than 20 grams a day, less than what is in a single apple. Despite early and persistent condemnation by nutritionists and physicians, these diets have been shown to work without being dangerous. As I related earlier, I lost 25 pounds in six weeks when I was on it. That is the rule, not the exception.

These diets have few long-term risks. They can trigger gout, a painful inflammation of one or more joints, constipation, and a few other minor issues. It is recommended to take a multivitamin because of the lack of fruit and vegetables in the diet. A rare person (and I was one) can develop dangerously high cholesterol levels, but overall, it is a reasonably safe way to lose weight.

Over time, the Atkins Diet has allowed for more fruit and vegetables, but not a lot. Once you have progressed on the diet, you can start eating other foods with carbs, but only in small amounts. The ketogenic diet is like the original Atkins Diet. It stresses more fat and less protein, but it is so similar that I think of it as the same as the Atkins diet.

I do sometimes recommend these diets for patients who have been discouraged by other diets, especially if they have significant weight to lose. The ketogenic diet is reliable and fast. If they stick to it, they can easily lose 20 pounds in the first month. But I don't like these diets for the long term. First, there is no reason to be that restrictive. You can lose weight, though maybe not as fast, if you eat fruits, vegetables, beans, and nuts. This is more healthy, since these foods have health benefits. While not proven to be harmful, I still don't think it is a great idea to eat meat and cheese and eggs in sizable amounts, indefinitely. But even if you wanted to eat that way forever, almost no one does. They tire of eating with such little variety, and if you stick it out, and lose all the weight you plan to lose, then what? As with the diets I mentioned earlier, you have not learned anything. You will probably just go back to what you did before. You might try to moderate your carb intake, but you know how difficult it is to moderate.

Since I feel The Three Rules is the best solution, I don't talk much to patients about the very low-carb diets. But when I do, I recommend that they start the ketogenic diet for a brief time and move to The Three Rules. They gain confidence from the rapid weight loss, and they see with their own eyes how sugar is harmful. After changing to The Three Rules, people learn how to eat a healthy diet, lose weight, and keep it off forever.

Low Glycemic Diets

Soon after it became obvious that the Atkins Diet and similar very low-carb diets caused weight loss, many related diets were created. Most of these were lumped together as "modified Atkins Diets," and you will still hear the term. In my experience, *The South Beach Diet*, by Arthur Agatston, MD, is the most important of them. I followed the diet myself off and on for many years and found it to be less restrictive and more enjoy-able than the Atkins Diet. I lost weight, perhaps not as fast as with Atkins, but fast enough, and I kept the weight off—when I stuck to it.

All the diets in this category look at the glycemic index and to a lesser extent the glycemic load. As you recall, the glycemic index refers to how much your blood glucose rises after eating something that contains 50 grams of carbohydrate. Foods that have added sugar and processed, re-fined carbohydrates usually score high on the glycemic index. Proteins and fats are zero, having little or no effect on glucose in the blood. Most fruits and vegetables are low. Glycemic load takes into account how much you are eating at a time, roughly equivalent to a serving size on the package. (We all know that we usually eat more than the serving size listed.)

We lose weight when we don't eat the high glycemic foods, or at least we don't gain weight when we eat them. The foods that are the worst have both a high glycemic index and glycemic load. These foods, such as potatoes, are densely packed with carbs, so that one serving gives you a large amount, often more than the 50 grams, and gram for gram, those carbs raise your sugar significantly.

The South Beach Diet and other similar diet books explain the glycemic index and guide you to the foods okay to eat. But they can be complex to follow. I have not read all the books, but *The South Beach Diet* allows some foods in the later phases of the diet that are not allowed early on. There are charts and tables explaining what you can eat and when, and you can do an internet search to find where a certain food falls on the diet. Most people I know, myself included, do not want to memorize tables or carry notes when they grocery shop or eat out.

These diets also allow certain foods in small quantities. For example, during phase 2 of the South Beach Diet, you might have a serving of bread. Well, that sounds a lot like eating in moderation. If I could eat in moderation, or stop after eating one dinner roll every time, I would never have had a weight problem. Allowing small amounts of certain foods at different times of the diet sounds great—more variety, more of what we like. But it also allows us to play mind games with ourselves. "I can have one roll. Well, that was a small roll, I will have half of another." Then you are finding it difficult to stop.

The low glycemic diets work, and in a sense, The Three Rules is a low glycemic diet. But The Rules avoids the pitfalls of the South Beach and similar diets. I feel that it is better to have a few rules, even if they prohibit categories of food entirely, than to allow some foods in moderation, in a difficult to remember system. Using the analogy of alcohol again, it is like allowing an alcoholic a single 12 ounce bottle of light beer. It may seem more harsh to prohibit all alcohol, but it works. Yes, the Three Rules absolutely prohibits foods with added sugar. But if you cut out most but not all food with added sugar, you will be frustrated and perhaps not successful in your goal of weight loss and keeping it off. Nothing bothered me more in my days of dieting than giving up most of what I liked, yet still not being successful.

Medications and Surgery

When you cannot do something on your own, it is smart to ask for help.

Most overweight people have tried to lose weight on their own at least once and many have had at least some success. Despite extreme effort, some people still cannot lose weight, and they ask their doctor for help. I see patients all the time asking for medications or other interventions such as surgery. There is a stigma attached to medications and surgery, but there shouldn't be. Why is treatment for obesity somehow wrong, yet medication for cholesterol, or surgery for a hernia is not? There are many medical conditions that cannot be managed without medication or surgery.

That said, if possible, it is usually preferable to manage weight on your own. You achieve a sense of accomplishment leading to more lasting success; You avoid the risks inherent to all medications and all surgery. And you save money, though that is a minor issue, since losing weight by any method, even surgery, likely saves money in the long run. I do not prescribe medications or refer for surgery often, but I understand the benefits in some cases. I hope that you try the Three Rules, rather than go immediately to medications or surgery, but it is worth knowing what else is out there for people with a weight problem.

Weight-Loss Medications

The medications on the market today have some benefit and are generally safe.[18] Most are indicated for short-term use, but a few can be taken long-term. Physicians differ in their prescribing of weight-loss medications and how often, and I rarely prescribe them.

---

[18] While writing this book, Belviq, one of the most popular medications, was taken off the market because of a concern regarding cancer risk.

In short-term studies, you can expect a 5% weight loss.[19] That would mean if you weigh 200 pounds and you are obese, you would lose 10 pounds in 6-12 months. That is fine, but with adherence to a diet such as The Three Rules, a 200-pound person who is 50 pounds overweight could easily lose 25-30 pounds or more in that time frame. With medications, some people lose over 5%, but others lose less. In long-term studies, the weight loss is not usually progressive, with weight loss often slowing and reaching a plateau, even if you stay on the medication.

Besides the unimpressive weight loss, there are other reasons I don't use these medications often. There are always risks to them, though the approved ones seem to be reasonably safe. There is also a financial cost, and many insurance plans don't cover weight loss drugs, and when they do, there is usually a significant copay. The cost of the drug is far more than the cost of a gym membership or any new foods you would buy with a healthy diet plan.

The biggest reason I don't much like these medications is the same reason I don't like the meal replacement plans. You have not learned anything while taking weight loss drugs. When you stop the medication, the weight comes right back on. Do you want to stay on a medication forever to preserve a 10 pound weight loss? Staying on a diet with a few rules is better than taking a medication forever. When you stop the drug, you will almost certainly go back to your previous eating habits, because you did not intentionally change much about your eating when you were on the medication.

If you start by changing your eating habits, with The Three Rules, or any diet for that matter, you avoid medications, you learn something, and you can lose weight. If you stick to the new lifestyle, you will keep the weight off.

---

[19] Khera, R., et al (2016). Association of Pharmacological Treatments for Obesity With Weight Loss and Adverse Events. *JAMA, 315*(22), 2424. https://doi.org/10.1001/jama.2016.7602

Bariatric Surgery

Bariatric surgery refers to the various surgical techniques designed to produce significant, sustained weight loss. I will not get into the details of the various surgeries, and I do not want to make specific recommendations of when you should consider bariatric surgery. I will discuss the benefits and risks of the surgery in general.

After bariatric surgery, people lose weight, a lot of weight. Studies show that obese people can often lose 100 pounds or more with certain surgical techniques. As a percentage of total weight, 25% weight loss is common. You probably have seen people who have lost more than that. Surgery can reverse diabetes, sleep apnea, hypertension, and other conditions. Overall survival and quality of life both improve in most studies. Over time, some weight is regained, but not usually all the weight.

So what are the downsides? Surgery has risks, with the overall risks varying by surgery type. There is a risk of death from the surgery itself, with the 30 day mortality being between 0.2% and 0.5% in most studies. The overall complication rate is higher, but most surgical complications are successfully managed. Don't forget though that there is a significant mortality and morbidity risk from remaining obese. The life expectancy of the obese who do not lose weight is much higher than those who lose the weight.

Comparing the benefits and risks of obesity surgery is complex. Those who lose weight on their own, as you will if you follow The Three Rules, do so with negligible risk. Without a good plan, though, most people are unsuccessful on their own. There is another concept regarding surgical risk that is often not considered. Let's say that a study showed that a surgery has a 1% mortality risk at 30 days, but the risk of dying without surgery is 2% at 10 years. (These are not the actual numbers with bariatric surgery, but the numbers are close enough for this example to help.) The 1% risk is right up front. If you are in that 1%, that is it, you are gone. If you don't have surgery and you are in the 2% group who dies in the next 10 years, at least on average you have several years of living. So the overall death risk is higher without surgery in this example, but you may have a better overall likelihood of living several years.

Aside from surgical risks, a major downside of bariatric surgery is that it will change your eating. Of course, that is part of the upside. But you will be completely unable to eat certain foods. You may get diarrhea, bloating, or vomiting if you eat what you shouldn't. You may be at risk for anemia and vitamin deficiencies, and certain medications need to be avoided. Lastly, some people regain significant amounts of weight, years after the surgery.

All that said, there are some excellent reasons to have bariatric surgery. If your doctor thinks you should have surgery, talk it over with them carefully, and definitely consider it. But, if you have not yet put all your effort into losing weight without surgery, I would recommend trying that first. In the next section, you will learn why I feel The Three Rules is the best solution to your weight problem.

Part 3: The Three Rules—the Best Solution

---

*Why should others believe the promises I make to them, if I do not
keep the promises I make to myself?*

Rules can have a negative connotation. We often learn to resent
the rules imposed on us by our parents, our teachers, and our
bosses. Yet to keep some level of order, we need some rules. It
is helpful to have rules and principles to live by. The Three Rules to Lose
Weight and Keep It Off Forever is a set of rules of eating that we impose
on ourselves. If you don't like the word "rules," call them "promises to
yourself."

The critical concept is eating with intent. Eating and drinking are perhaps the most important actions of any animal's daily life, including ours.
In today's world, food and water are so plentiful, we don't give it a
thought. We need to eat with intent, meaning we need to think about
what we are eating. An animal in the wild, and humans before us, did not
have this luxury. To survive, we had to eat virtually everything we encountered, Now, rarely hungry, we should think about everything we eat.
Do I want to eat from a bowl of candy? Do I want to keep Doritos in
the house and eat them any time I want? Should I eat the apple in the
fridge? It is a helpful concept for all of what we do. Do everything, including eating, with intent.

We have discussed some key points of the diet and I will now go over
the actual Rules. I will show you that while the Rules require effort, you
will be able to live a normal, happy life. Losing weight and keeping it off,
the goal of The Three Rules, will give you greater health, help prevent
disease, improve your quality of life, and allow you to be more active and
take part in more rewarding activities as you get older.

The Rules will change how you eat, but you will still be able to eat. You will not be hungry, will have many options, and will be able to travel and eat at restaurants with little difficulty. Yesterday was Thanksgiving. I had turkey, ham, brussels sprouts, green beans, beet hummus with vegetables (very good, my niece made it), Greek salad, and assorted cheeses. I did not eat the pumpkin cheesecake or mashed potatoes. It was a good Thanksgiving with my family, and I did not feel deprived. I also was one of the few people who did not complain of feeling tired and bloated after.

The Rules are all about what to *remove* from your diet. There is not a single food that causes weight loss. On the web, there are ads for "fat-burning foods" or "cardiologist says this food will cause weight loss." Not true. All diets work by removing something from what you normally eat—calories, carbs, sugars, fats, whatever. The Three Rules involves removing what I call **bad carbs** from your diet. Another term I will use for bad carbs is **junk food**. There are various definitions of junk food, but when I use it, I mean bad carbs.

There are three categories of **bad carbs**, and in The Three Rules, you remove all of them. When you do that, you have to eat something. So you eat good carbs, proteins, and fats. These good foods are not the cause of the weight loss. They are what you eat after removing the fattening foods. A steak does not cause weight loss, but it allows for the weight loss that occurs after removing the four donuts from your diet.

You have heard The Rules earlier in the book to some extent, but we have to be clear on exactly what The Rules means. The Rules are simple, but they are strict. If you generally follow The Rules, but not closely enough, you may succeed, but you may not. Following any diet only partially often leads to giving up some of what you like *and* failing in your ultimate goal of weight loss. This causes frustration, and you will probably quit the diet. If you are strict, The Rules plan works.

The Three Rules are not perfect. It would be nice if every single food group could be absolutely good or absolutely bad. That is not how nature is. Fortunately there are only a few foods in this gray area. I avoid these. Why risk it? There are so many other choices. Two examples of gray area foods are whole grain flour and brown rice. Neither one fits perfectly into a Rule. I don't eat either. Both are uncommon enough and easily avoided. Why ruin a diet on a few avoidable foods?

Dieters find it difficult to accept that the "All or None" approach works best. When starting The Three Rules, it seems hard to believe that I am asking you to give up bread, sugar, potatoes, or something else completely, 100%. In the first few days or weeks of the plan, it is difficult. You are used to eating a piece of candy, or a roll with dinner. But giving it up completely is far easier than having a little. I repeat it over and over, because it is true. You would never recommend to a reformed alcoholic to have a small beer or to treat themselves to a shot of tequila on a holiday. One drink won't hurt them, but they cannot stop at one drink. A cookie won't hurt me, but I cannot stop at one cookie. It is the same thing. I do not believe in cheat days or treats. An occasional treat becomes a daily treat which is the same as a habit.

All or None is the scariest part of the Three Rules and also its greatest strength. Committing to it is daunting, but you will succeed. If a person with an addiction commits to conquering alcohol or drugs, they give them up completely. If they do that, they are certain to succeed. If you give up completely the bad carbs outlawed by the Three Rules, your success is nearly certain.

I will go over each Rule and common issues that people have when implementing it. The Rules sound straightforward, and they are. But foods are not always simple in themselves. We eat foods with many components. Foods are marketed to sound healthy, and food labels do not always tell the complete picture.

I hope you will agree with me that The Rules are simpler and easier than guidelines, charts, counting and measuring. That carbs are easier to control than hunger. That giving up some groups of foods is easier than cutting back on all food. In the later sections, you will learn a few issues specific to keeping weight off forever. I will help with some tricks, pointers, and pitfalls and will discuss other aspects of eating and lifestyle that might apply. You will realize that as with anything, even an excellent plan has downsides. I hope and expect that you will realize that if you follow The Three Rules, the benefits greatly outweigh these negatives.

Rule One: Do Not Eat Food With Added Sugar

Sugar has been called the new smoking. I don't know if it's that bad, but it's bad.

I have discussed why sugar causes weight gain. When we eat sugar, our blood glucose rises, triggering the rise in fat-storing hormones, especially insulin. Different foods have this effect to varying degrees. This is the glycemic index and glycemic load. Added sugar raises our blood sugar the most, and the more you eat, the worse it is. But as you know, moderation and limiting yourself to a little of something is very difficult. Don't eat any.

General Concepts And Common Foods

There is sugar in fruit, vegetables, beans, nuts, and dairy. This has no bearing on Rule 1. We are talking about sugar added to the otherwise healthy good carbs, protein, and fat in your food. I will say it many times, but here it is. Sugar that is put into a food product or a dish you make at home will rapidly raise your blood glucose and make it easy to gain weight and difficult to lose it. Don't eat it if sugar is added. Read the ingredients section of the food label. You can look at the Nutrition Facts section and see that there may be grams of sugar in foods like mixed nuts, but unless there is sugar added, eat it.

Most of the foods off limits because of Rule 1 are obvious. At a store, foods are packaged and processed, and they report the sugar on the label. But you have to look carefully. Sugar has many names: corn syrup, evaporated cane juice, rice syrup, dextrose, sucrose, glucose, fruit juice concentrate, maltodextrin, molasses, and many more.[20] I was tempted to list all the ones I could find, but it became ridiculous. Instead, I have referenced in the footnote the University Of California website for more details. Some types of sugar may be a little better than others, but for me,

---

[20] https://sugarscience.ucsf.edu/hidden-in-plain-sight/web#.XeJajJNKi8U

an All or None eater, it only works if you avoid all of it. When in doubt regarding an ingredient, look it up.

Be wary of seemingly healthy foods, like granola. Most granola is a mixture of a few nuts, processed oats (against Rule 2) and a sugar-sweetener, sometimes honey. Honey is just dissolved sugar made by bees rather than humans. I am not sure how granola ever became considered healthy. It may have a few benefits, but it definitely will raise your blood sugar. Trail mix is another example. There is often granola, sugar-sweetened fruit, and sometimes even candy. Just because someone says that a food is healthy, it doesn't mean it won't make you fat.

If you are making the food at home, it is easier to know what is off limits, since you are adding the sugar yourself—like cookies, pastries, sweetened sauces, and candy. But you also need to think about some sweeteners that don't sound like sugar. Adding corn syrup to your Christmas cookies is the same as adding sugar.

It is more difficult to follow Rule 1 when someone else is making your food, and you do not see the labels, such as in restaurants. Many restaurants now list ingredients. That is not quite as trustworthy as a packaged product's label, but it is pretty good. Most of the hidden sugar in restaurants is in the sauces and dressings. Don't be afraid to ask the wait staff if there is sugar added. If they are not sure, or you don't trust the answer, put it on the side. Usually a quick taste will tell you if there is significant sugar added, but not always. If you want to be strict, get a dish at a restaurant where it is obviously free of added sugars: most meat, chicken, and fish dishes can be made with no sweetened sauces. For salads, bleu cheese, vinaigrettes, and oil and vinegar are usually safe.

- **Read every label's ingredient list.**
- **Confirm that there is no added sugar.**
- **Double-check that there is no added sugar by a different name.**

Can I Eat Any Sugar?

Once you know the Rule, there really is nothing to understanding it. Don't eat food with added sugar. But that does not mean that you don't eat any sugar. Because we know that sugar is a component of so many foods, people still get it wrong all the time. When I tell people this Rule, they ask, "You don't eat any sugar?" I do eat sugar. I eat the sugar in most natural foods—fruit, vegetables, beans, nuts, and dairy. Just because a food is natural does not mean it is healthy or good for this diet, but the sugars in most natural foods are fine. Almost all fruits have sugar, and almost all fruits are fine on this diet. I eat at least three servings of fruit a day—apples, oranges, grapefruit, berries, whatever. Most of these fruits are sweet, not as sweet as candy, but sweet enough. And, if you don't eat sugar-sweetened foods, everything else tastes sweeter than it did before.

The key to this Rule is to read every label of every food you eat. Pay little attention to the grams of sugar in the "Nutrition Facts." If apples had labels, they would list about 20 grams of sugar. This is not added sugar. Some labels list added sugar grams, which is helpful, and for The Three Rules, it should be zero. (A bottle of Mountain Dew has 77 grams of added sugar, which is the same as 19 of the white packets.) What difference does it make if the sugar is added or in the food naturally? Again, it comes down to glycemic index, how much your blood glucose rises after eating the food. The main sugar in most fruit is fructose. At the levels in fruit, combined with the fiber in the fruit, your blood sugar doesn't rise much, and you cannot efficiently store fat. High fructose corn syrup is different, since it has so much fructose and glucose, it overwhelms your body. Glucose rises fast and you can store fat easily. I am not even going to get into the other harmful effects of this food additive.

Many foods have no added sugar, yet they have grams of sugar listed on the label. These are all fine to eat: milk, yogurt, nuts, vegetables, beans, canned tomatoes, some tomato sauces, salad dressings, and many more. A perfect example is the wonderful Costco plain non-fat Greek yogurt, in which there are 7 grams of carbohydrate and 4 grams of sugar per serving. In the ingredients, there is only milk. There is no sugar *added*. In the left column, you see that there are 4 grams of sugars. That is all lactose. You can (and should) eat this on The Three Rules plan. If you are wondering, I eat it with frozen berries for breakfast at work, nearly every day. You put the yogurt and berries in a food storage container the night before and it is perfect by morning. I sometimes add cinnamon or cocoa powder for a unique taste. While the fruit has fructose and the yogurt has lactose, neither raises blood glucose or fat-storing hormones much.

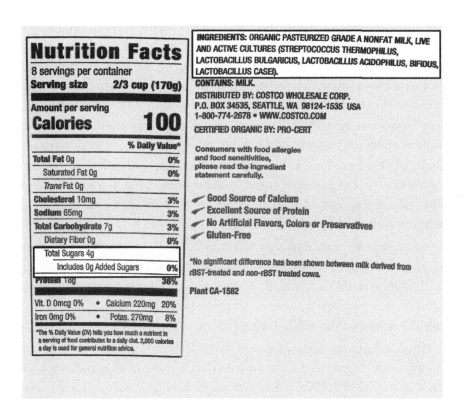

In case you are wondering, beans and nuts have almost no effect on blood glucose because of the fiber content and the type of sugar and starch in it. If you stick to The Rules, even high calorie nuts will allow for weight loss.

- **Sugar in all its forms should not be in the ingredients.**
- **Grams of sugar in the Nutrition Facts do not matter, as long as there is no added sugar.**

If It's Not Sweet, Can I Eat It?

You might by surprised by some foods that have added sugar. Diced tomatoes, canned beans, and other canned vegetables will sometimes have added sugar in the processing. Again, most vegetables and all beans have grams of sugar, but the fiber prevents your glucose from rising quickly in your blood. Make sure there is no added sugar in the can you are buying. Even savory sauces can have sugar added. Just a few weeks ago, a patient told me he was not succeeding on the diet. He was eating a lot of tomato sauce. I asked him if there was sugar added, and he said he did not know. He had given up so many foods but had not lost weight. That is frustrating for him, but he was not reading the labels. I don't know if there was sugar added in his sauce, but if he was not reading labels, he may have been eating a lot of added sugar. Condiments are also common sources of hidden sugar. Ketchup has about 3 grams of added sugar per tablespoon. Most people use far more than one tablespoon of ketchup, so that sugar adds up.

Many snack foods that are not sweet break Rule 1. Graham crackers are sweet enough to know that they are against the Rule. Would you think Rold Gold pretzels have added sugar? Read the label—corn syrup! There is just no way to know without reading the label. (Pretzels are also against Rule 2 because of the refined wheat in it.)

Protein bars are notorious. Clif Bars, PowerBars, and Snickers bars all have over 20 grams of sugar added. That is not counting the other bad carbs in them. There are some low sugar bars, but very few have zero sugar added. Don't assume that if a bar is labeled "low sugar" that you can eat it. Low is not zero. Would 5 grams of added sugar in a protein bar derail your diet? Almost certainly not. But 5 grams several times a day might. Eating low sugar foods in small amounts involves eating in moderation. As I say again and again, most of us cannot eat in moderation. I am best off choosing a snack with zero added sugar. Then I don't think about it. I snack on nuts, fruit, beef jerky (some have sugar added), cheese, and many other foods. I don't find it difficult to survive. Another problem is that store-bought snacks usually have refined carbs, which are against Rule 2.

- **Most snack foods and protein bars have added sugar.**
- **Many sauces, even the savory ones, have added sugar.**

Final Point On Rule 1

Rule 1 simply means giving up foods with added sugar. That really is not hard to follow in the long run, but it can be tough when you start out. It was a change for me to pay attention to sugar and to read every label. But once you get in the habit, it is rather easy. We tend to eat the same foods over and over. Most products are obvious and you don't need to read the labels: Candy, doughnuts, cookies—obviously out. For other things, I don't have to read many labels at all anymore, since I stay with the same brands for my staple foods. I read the label for any new product I eat. A product similar to one I normally eat may have unexpected added sugar, but it may also have something against Rule 2 or 3. Don't forget that there are two more Rules. All Three Rules need to be observed.

Rule Two: Do Not Eat Food With Processed
And Refined Carbohydrates

Processing and refining may be good in some settings, but not when it comes to eating.

This Rule is more difficult to explain and more difficult to follow than Rule 1. I even have had some difficulty coming up with the wording. First, I used only "processed" but that seemed to imply that even processing fruit into dried fruit, peanuts into peanut butter, or milk into yogurt somehow raised the glycemic index and made them against the Rules. I also tried "refined" but that was also somewhat vague, and refining somehow sounds like a good thing. Now I use both words, knowing that it is not a simple rule to understand without further explanation. Processing means that something was done to the natural food before we eat it. When I use the word "refine," I mean that something good was changed or removed from the food. Note that none of this applies to foods such as meats and fats that have no carbohydrates. Any form of meat or oil is fine.

The problem with processed, refined carbs is that they raise your blood glucose quickly, reflected in the glycemic index. Most natural foods like nuts, beans, fruit, vegetables, and most whole grains won't raise blood sugar high enough to interfere with weight loss. Processed and refined foods like flour and white rice will. The biggest culprit in this category by far are the processed wheat products—bread, pasta, crackers, other snack foods, pastries, cookies, and breakfast cereal. When the bran and fiber are removed from wheat, the glycemic index skyrockets. (This has nothing to do with gluten—gluten may affect some people, but it is a protein and is not relevant in this diet.) Most of these products also have added sugar, so they are doubly bad, against two of the Three Rules.

Not all processed foods are off limits. Food without carbs, such as processed meats, are fine with The Three Rules Plan. (There may be other health issues, but that is a topic for another book.) Some processed foods with carbohydrates are also fine for The Three Rules. Taking fruit, vegetables, nuts, and beans, and chopping them up or mashing them does not significantly change the glycemic index, even though they are processed in one sense of the word. Chopping and mashing fruit is fine, but removing fiber and pulp leaves only the sugars and raises the glycemic index. A popular dish now is mashed cauliflower. This is the same for your body as eating whole cauliflower. (Your stomach mashes in much the same way.) Peanut and other nut butters are just mashed nuts and since nuts are good, then nut butter is also good. You must read the label because many nut butters and mashed fruit products have added sugars or other ingredients you want to avoid.

This brings us to one of the "gray area" foods I was talking about. My wife has pointed out to me many times over the years that not everything is black and white. I know that, but my brain has trouble accepting it. I told you that the Three Rules is not perfect—nothing is. Richard Carlson taught that we should "make peace with imperfection," and I am working on it. I have accepted that grains are in this category. If you eat unprocessed whole grains other than rice (we will talk about rice later), the glycemic index is low and you can eat it. But if you grind it up fine enough, as in flour, then even if unrefined, your body digests and absorbs the carbs rapidly, your glucose rises, and you can easily gain weight. In other words, the glycemic index goes up when you make flour from grain. We will talk about whole grains in the next chapter and again with Rule 3. **For now, just know that all flour made from grain is against Rule 2.**

Most people find that Rule 2 is the hardest of The Rules to follow when they start off. We do not go into withdrawals when we stop eating these foods, we just have habits of eating bread, cereal, pasta, and refined-wheat products, and making these foods is easy and quick. Many of my patients cannot conceive of starting the day without cereal or toast. But, what is wrong with eggs, yogurt, cottage cheese, fruit, ham, or smoked salmon for breakfast? Is it suffering to eat a salad with chicken, tuna lettuce wraps, vegetables and peanut butter, or fruit and cheese for lunch? Is steak and salad, chicken and brussels sprouts, or salmon and green beans so bad for dinner? Once you go a few weeks, you will have no trouble finding a variety of foods to eat.

Wheat, Flour, And Corn Products

After sugar, the most significant bad carbs in our diet are from wheat and corn, typically in bread, pasta, cereal, snack foods, and pastries. Refining whole grains means removing the bran and germ layers, the parts of the grain with fiber, and fiber blunts the rise in glucose. When these layers are removed, it requires even more of the remaining, high-glycemic parts of the grain to make bread or whatever product you are making. So you eat none of the glucose blunting part and more of the glucose raising part.

If a food, such as wheat, is high in carbs to begin with, the worse it is with processing. Whole wheat kernels do not affect blood sugar much. Grinding the wheat and removing the bran and fiber causes the blood sugar to go way up. But it turns out that whole grain flour and the similar wholemeal flour have nearly as high a glycemic index, despite having none of the bran and fiber removed. This is because there is so much starch in wheat and other grains that when the particles are small enough, we can digest a significant amount of starch.

Nearly all grains can be processed into flour. Besides the usual wheat flour, you will find rye, barley, and less commonly, millet and amaranth. These may be slightly better than wheat flour, but the difference is not enough to help your diet. The rise in the popularity of gluten-free products has led to potato and rice flours, just about the worst foods for a low glycemic diet. If it is a gluten-free bakery product, it is likely to be bad for any weight loss plan. Nuts have so little starch and carbohydrate that even grinding it into flour or butter has a minor effect. That is why almond and other nut flours are fine and all flour from grain is off limits.

Bread is one of the most difficult things for me to avoid—I grew up on bagels. I don't know anyone who doesn't like bread. It is also very convenient—you can make a lunch or dinner in one minute with bread and lunchmeat. You can make breakfast with two pieces of bread and a toaster. But bread is a major contributor to our weight problems. White bread has a glycemic index close to 100, as high as eating pure glucose. In fact, the glycemic index of white bread is higher than eating an equivalent amount of table sugar. It is often used as a standard for the highest possible glycemic index, against which other foods are tested. As we just discussed, whole wheat or whole grain bread is not much better. Some breads in stores have a modest glycemic index, but they are packed with carbs, meaning that you reach the 50 gram limit quickly. Since we cannot moderate very well, we overeat these breads and ruin our diet. You must avoid all bread if you want to be successful.

Snack foods we eat are usually made from refined wheat and corn, so you probably can figure out that most such products are forbidden by Rule 2. When in doubt, reading the labels helps. Ritz Crackers, my favorite in the past, have ground wheat, and the label says "wheat flour" right on it. But you have to be careful. The Triscuit label says, "whole grain wheat," and the Wheat Thins label says, "whole grain wheat flour." There may be differences in how the wheat is processed in the three wonderful snacks, but that doesn't matter. They all have wheat flour and all must be avoided. All three also have sugar and break Rule 1. I don't even bother reading labels of crackers and cookies. Virtually all break Rule 1, Rule 2, or both. Don't eat them.

Breakfast cereal is also a very easy meal to prepare. But most cereal is just chopped up bread or refined corn, soaked in some sweetener or other. When I mention the problems with cereal, people sometimes are crestfallen. Yes, most of us like cereal. It is tasty, simple to prepare, and it reminds us of childhood. I would be surprised if I have eaten fewer than 500 bowls of Cap'n Crunch cereal. But even the non-sweet varieties like Cheerios or Shredded Wheat are very high on the glycemic index and will ruin almost any diet. Hot cereals like Cream of Wheat or Malt-O-Meal are the same as any cold cereals. All cereal is against the rules because of the glycemic index and load, and like pasta, we usually eat far more than a single serving. Put 3/4 cup cereal into a bowl and see if that is what you normally eat for breakfast.

Pasta is another staple of the American diet. But it is refined wheat with a few other ingredients. It is especially harmful if you are trying to lose weight. The glycemic index is not all that high, but the serving size is small, and we easily reach the 50 grams of glycemic index and usually double it with a typical meal. That is not even counting the junk we often put on the pasta. If you could stick to a 2 ounce (1/8 of a box) of spaghetti and put no bad carbs on it, you would not gain weight. You might even lose weight. But no one does that. Pasta is off limits on The Three Rules.

Most corn products are just as bad as wheat. These include tortillas, cornbread, polenta, grits and others. Many of these dishes have sugar added, but even without it, they are against Rule 2 because they are processed and refined. Refined corn significantly contributes to obesity, but even unrefined corn is problematic because it is starchy, and corn is against Rule 3.

After just a few days on the Three Rules plan, it will be obvious that most snack foods and all bread are off limits. Reading the label will prove it, but be careful. Your default assumption should be not to eat it. Very few snack foods, despite what the label implies, have whole grains that have not been processed. If it lists whole wheat berries, or another whole grain, and it says unrefined or unprocessed on the package, and I can see the unprocessed, unrefined, whole grain in the food, then I might eat it. There are a few snack bars at health foods stores that might fit in this category. But if you cannot see the whole grain, then assume it is processed and refined. I have said before in this book, and say it every day with patients, "Don't ruin your plans with dieting over something that isn't all that good to begin with." Wheat Thins are good, but would you want to sabotage your weight control over it? Would you want to waste all that hard work on a mediocre protein bar? If I go off the diet, give me something better than that, say a Sourdough Jack Burger.

- **Do not eat bread or flour from wheat or any grain.**
- **Do not eat any food made from ground wheat or other grains.**
- **Do not eat corn products.**

Oats

Oats are difficult. As we will learn in Rule 3, all grains have starches that are turned into glucose. *Unrefined* oats have mostly resistant starches, meaning that we do not digest them easily into glucose. Most people can eat unrefined oats and still lose weight and keep it off. The principal problem with oats is when it is made into quick or instant oatmeal, or granola. Unrefined oats and other grains are called groats, so unprocessed oats are oat groats. I put oat groats and barley in the same food category, because they have similar effects on blood glucose, and after cooking they are very similar in taste and use in foods.

When I last lost weight, I did not eat any grains, but now I know that most people can eat unprocessed whole grains (other than corn and rice) and still lose weight. Oat groats are not, however, what you eat when you have oatmeal or granola.

Unprocessed oats can take as long as an hour or more to make. Steel-cut oats is groats, chopped into a few pieces, and is nearly equivalent to the groats. Rolled oats and instant oats are much more refined and can be cooked in a few minutes. The glycemic index rises in processing and refining, with instant oatmeal being about 50% higher than steel-cut oats. I stick to The Rules strictly, so I don't eat any oats except groats and steel-cut. I make a large batch of oat groats or barley and add it to yogurt and other foods. It adds texture and tastes great, far better than the packages of instant oatmeal.

While there are some issues with unprocessed whole grains, they are not the major problem. Quick or instant oatmeal is refined and processed and against The Rules. If your oatmeal was made in a few minutes, it was refined and processed and will interfere with your diet plan. A large bowl of instant oatmeal in the morning ruins lots of diets, even if you don't add the maple syrup and brown sugar.

- **Don't eat oatmeal unless it is groats or steel-cut.**

Rice

White rice, which is refined and processed, is definitely against Rule 2. It has a high glycemic index, and we eat it in excess all the time. At an Asian restaurant, you will see people pile white rice on their plates. Even if they choose the entrée without the sweet sauce, their blood glucose and weight will jump. White rice will ruin your diet, unless you can eat in insignificant amounts. As always, All or None is easier than moderation.

We usually eat the rice in sushi in limited amounts, and some people can lose weight eating it, just as some people can eat a square of chocolate a day. Since I don't do well with even a little of something against The Rules, I don't eat sushi. I recommend completely avoiding rice, for the same reasons that everything against the Rules should be avoided entirely.

Parboiled Rice or converted rice is processed in a way that removes some of the starch and carbohydrates, and it has a lower glycemic index than white rice. But it is still too high on the glycemic load because it is packed with carbs, and you reach the 50 grams of the glycemic index in no time. It is very difficult to moderate and like all processed, refined foods, it is against Rule 2.

Brown rice (starchy and discussed in the next section) is unprocessed and unrefined, but it has more digestible starches than most unrefined grains and has a high glycemic index and glycemic load. I have seen people substitute brown rice for white rice, then overeat it and end up ruining their diets. I consider all rice to be against the Rules.

Refined grains and the products made from them are high glycemic and difficult to moderate, addictive in some sense. I would not eat them at all, sticking completely to the All or None philosophy. It is too easy to keep going back to the bowl of rice, to keep going back to the all you can eat sushi. Even in small amounts, these foods can ruin diets. Worse, we cannot stop at even the small amounts.

- **Don't eat any rice.**

Juice and Refined Fruit Products

Processed and refined wheat causes much of the weight gain in this country. But processed and refined fruit doesn't help. Juice is refined in the terrible sense of the word. It has none of the fiber, pulp, and other components of the fruit or vegetable that slow glucose production.

The other problem with juice is that it takes about three oranges to make a cup of juice. We could easily drink a cup of juice in a few minutes, whereas eating three oranges would take time, and I have never eaten three oranges at one time. Our blood glucose rises faster and higher than it would if we just ate the fruit. Apple, grape, and most other juices are even more of a problem because even more of the fiber and pulp are removed. Many juices in the store have sugar added, making it even worse for your weight.

All fruit juice is against the Rules, and it is one of the worst things you can consume, nearly as bad as a soft drink. If you see fruit juice listed in the ingredients of a product, consider that fruit juice to be sugar. I don't think I need to tell you, but fruit rolls, fruit candy and all similar fruit products are against The Rules. They are processed and refined, and they usually have added sugar.

Some vegetable juices, like tomato and carrot juice, might be okay because the sugar content is so low to begin with, but I prefer to avoid all juice, so I don't have to think about it. I figure that there are nearly infinite things that I can eat and drink on this diet, and if I miss a few because the Rules are easier to follow this way, so be it.

I want to make a comment on smoothies. If you make them yourself in a blender or Vitamix, and you don't add any sugar, that is fine. I never have smoothies at a shop unless I am very confident that there is no sugar syrup or other sugar added and that the whole fruit is in the smoothie. Remember, if pulp and other fruit fiber is removed, then you are drinking juice. Stores may also add yogurt, peanut butter, and protein, all of which could be fine but could have sweeteners added. Be certain that there is no added sugar and that the whole fruit is in the drink.

I eat several servings of fruit a day. I love it. Eating an apple is more rewarding than apple juice. The same is true for all fruit and most vege-tables. It makes little sense to ruin your diet over something like juice or a smoothie, when the fruit is better and won't cause weight gain.

- **Don't drink juice.**
- **Don't eat refined fruit products.**

Milk and Dairy

It would be nice if Rule Two were perfectly black and white, with all refined foods being bad—it would be easier to remember. There are a few foods though that are fine to eat but are technically processed and refined. A stickler would say that dairy products such as cheese and yogurt are processed and refined, because fat and other constituents of milk might be removed in the processing. But none of what is removed makes a significant difference to your blood sugar or your weight. Milk and dairy products will not make you gain weight while you are on a diet like The Three Rules, and I recommend you eat dairy if you like it.

Multiple studies show that milk and most unsweetened dairy products have a low glycemic index and don't cause weight gain. Unsweetened Greek yogurt is especially good because of all the protein in it. There is no reason on this diet to avoid milk, cheese, or yogurt, whether or not there is fat in it. In fact, full-fat dairy products seem to have no ill effects, a fact shown in multiple recent studies. I guess I stick to the non-fat yogurt for two reasons. It is inexpensive at Costco, and as my wife reminds me, I still get hung up on what we learned in medical school, that all dairy fat is bad, which as we now know, it is not. So, my advice is to eat any unsweetened dairy you want. Most yogurt with fruit in it has added sugar, so be careful. Some yogurt will have other additives. We will talk about them later, but just know that some of them violate Rule 3.

As I mentioned earlier, a superb way to eat yogurt is to put it in a dish or travel container with frozen fruit, leaving it in the fridge overnight. Buying the yogurt and fruit in bulk is inexpensive. Frozen fruit has all the nutrition of fresh, is usually already washed, and never goes bad in the freezer. It is typically less than half the price of fresh.

- **Dairy is good, unless there is added sugar or other prohibited additives.**

Nut Milks and Other Replacement Milks

Replacement milks from beans or nuts such as soy, almond, coconut, cashew, macadamia and others are also allowed in The Three Rules. They are made by grinding the nuts or beans, adding water, and removing some byproducts. This is another case where some refining doesn't seem to make a difference.

I was drinking unsweetened almond milk for a long time before I even realized that it technically was refined by my definition. I looked into the various milks and even though some of the original nut is removed, the glycemic index doesn't change much from the index of the original form. Also, since a cup of the drink is mostly water, there are so few carbs in it that the glycemic load is negligible. For example, a cup of unsweetened almond milk has 1 gram of carbohydrate and no sugar. Remember that the glycemic index is calculated from 50 grams of carbohydrate, so 50 cups of almond milk would be needed. Obviously a cup of the drink doesn't make a difference. Would I prefer that The Three Rules were perfect and there were no "good" foods that technically violate the wording of the Rules? Yes. But nature and life are not perfect. If you want to be an absolute Three Rules purist, avoid all the replacement milks and stick with whole dairy milk. But over the years, I am getting better at making peace with imperfection, so I drink almond milk.

All the replacement milks listed above are fine. Do not drink rice milk. Most rice milk is made from white rice or rice flour, both highly refined. Some are chemically (enzymatically) processed and the starches are converted to sugars, even worse. The important thing is that the glycemic index of rice milk is much higher than regular milk or the nut "milks." A cup of rice milk has about 25 grams of carbohydrate, meaning that in contrast to almond milk, with its one gram of carbohydrate per cup, with rice milk, you are half-way to the 50 gram carb level of the glycemic index. Don't drink it.

Tofu is made by coagulating soy milk in much the same way that cheese is made from regular milk. In some health food stores, you will see non-dairy "cheese" made the same way from nuts and other beans. Just like dairy cheese, these are fine.

As always, you need to read the labels, if you drink any replacement milk or eat any of the cheese made from it. Most of the drinks at the store will have added sugar, and a few have prohibited food additives. (We will talk about food additives more in the Rule 3 section.) Obviously, sugar breaks Rule 1—no added sugar. I never drink soy or almond milk at a restaurant or coffee shop without reading the label. The coffee shops will usually let you see the package. But you will see that in most cases, sugar is added. If I want something to lighten my coffee at a coffee shop, I use milk or cream—I have never seen sugar added to these. Of course, whipped cream often has sugar added.

- **Unsweetened replacement milk from soy and nuts are fine.**
- **Do not drink rice milk.**

Alcohol

We all know that alcohol has significant risks to health and can definitely affect one's ability to lose weight. Alcohol is made from carbohydrates, so we need to talk about it in Rule 2. Alcohol's effect on health and weight is confusing and controversial. People have strong opinions on how much we should drink, how much is safe, and even the morality of drinking. I will try to stick with the facts, but my opinion may show through. Beer is against Rule 2 because it is refined grain—usually wheat or barley. Sweet drinks, including the sweet wines, have sugar added and are against Rule 1. Dry wine has sugar added, but it is all consumed by the yeast. Hard liquor, such as whiskey or vodka, has no carbs and is within the Rules.

Many studies show that alcohol in moderation can lower the risk of heart disease. In larger quantities, alcohol is clearly harmful, increasing the risk of liver disease, heart problems, stroke, and cancer. We all know of the dangers of acute intoxication. Many people cannot consume any alcohol without risking binging or becoming addicted. I will put all that aside for now and discuss the effects of alcohol on a carbohydrate-based diet.

Alcohol has variable effects on glucose metabolism, depending on the person and when they drink it. An important factor is what type of alcoholic drink you consume. I am confident of one thing—beer contributes to weight gain, presumably by raising glucose[21], and most heavy beer drinkers I know are overweight or obese. Studies are less conclusive with dry wine and spirits, though alcohol in any form in high quantities seems to raise blood sugar for some people.[22]

If you want to lose weight, you should not drink beer or sweet wine. Too much dry wine or liquor may sabotage some people's diet plans, and possibly your life plans. If you want to drink dry wine or liquor, you are likely fine with regard to The Three Rules, but if you cannot drink in moderation, you have three problems. First, you may not lose weight because of the effects of alcohol on your metabolism. Second, you are more likely to make poor food choices, not to mention many other poor choices. And third, you probably should abstain from alcohol completely, since if you cannot drink in moderation, you by definition have an alcohol problem.

- **Do not drink beer.**
- **Do not drink sweet wine.**
- **Dry wine and liquor are within The Rules, but be careful, for many reasons.**

---

[21] Sluik, D., et al (2016). Contributors to dietary glycaemic index and glycaemic load in the Netherlands: the role of beer. *British Journal of Nutrition*, *115*(7), 1218–1225. https://doi.org/10.1017/s0007114516000052

[22] Hätönen, K. A., et al (2012). Modifying effects of alcohol on the postprandial glucose and insulin responses in healthy subjects. *The American Journal of Clinical Nutrition*, *96*(1), 44–49. https://doi.org/10.3945/ajcn.111.031682

Rule Three: Do Not Eat Starchy Vegetables Or Fruits, Especially Potatoes, Corn, And Rice

Put starch on your shirts—don't eat it.

Starch, as you recall from the initial chapters, is a carbohydrate molecule that is broken down into sugar. Many starches, especially that in potato, are digested quickly into glucose, causing all the problems with weight that we have discussed. We love potatoes and we eat a lot, in many forms. It is ironic, but the classic meat and potatoes diet causes more harm from the potatoes than the meat. If you eliminate potatoes from your diet, you have almost mastered this rule.

Do not get hung up on botanical terms. I used to be concerned about whether tomato was a fruit, whether grains are fruits, whether corn is a grain or a fruit or a vegetable. Who cares? I call all nuts "nuts," whether they are tree nuts, legumes, or something else. I call corn a vegetable in some settings and a grain or cereal in others. As far as this diet goes, it doesn't matter. Starchy is starchy and we should avoid it whether it is a starchy fruit, vegetable, grain, or a combination.

Not all starches are problematic. The starch in potato is easily digested and converted to glucose. Others are not easily digested and are called resistant starches. The list of foods that have a considerable amount of starch is long and most consist of resistant starches and don't matter to us. Beans and other legumes, squash, and nuts have mostly resistant starches, are great to eat, and I don't even think of these as starchy foods. For the purpose of the Rule, they are not starchy—we only care about the digestible starches, the ones that cause us to gain weight. Beans and nuts are good, and I eat them almost every day. Potatoes, sweet potatoes, corn, and rice have too much digestible starch; they are starchy and against Rule 3. A few foods are in a gray area, and have variable amounts of resistant and digestible starches, depending on how you eat them—bananas are the most significant.

In this chapter, we will go over the most important fruits and vegetables. I will elaborate more on grains, and I will talk about a few more food additives. But if all you take home is the fundamental point of Rule 3, you will do well. Do not eat potatoes, sweet potatoes, corn, or rice.

- **Beans, nuts, and most fruits and vegetables are good.**
- **Do not eat potatoes, sweet potatoes, corn, or rice.**

Potatoes

I love potatoes. I have found very few people who do not enjoy eating potatoes in one form or another. They are inexpensive and give us quick energy. Unfortunately, everything comes with a price. The potato has a high glycemic index because of its rapidly digestible starch and is the prototype of a starchy vegetable. It is very difficult to lose weight if you eat potatoes, even if you almost starve yourself the rest of the day.

Years ago, Americans could get by with a potato at dinner, because as we have discussed, our lives were different in what we ate and the energy we burned with normal activities. Meat and potatoes at dinner would sustain us. The meat gave us protein and fat, and the potato supplied all the carbs we needed. A few green vegetables and fruit once in a while, and we were good. Now we eat potatoes in multiple forms, all the time. Chips, fries, mashed, hash browns, baked, boiled—it doesn't matter. It is all high glycemic and bad for any diet. We were told long ago that it was what you put on a baked potato, such as sour cream or bacon, that caused the weight gain. That is not true, at least not now. With our current lives, it is the glucose generated from the potato itself.

Potatoes also act like an addictive substance. I am sure it is not truly addictive, like a drug, but once you get started, like so many tasty carbs, it is difficult to stop. Just like the old Lay's potato chip commercial told us, it is hard to eat just one. That is true with most forms of potato. I find it rather easy to have none, but not one. If you cannot give up potatoes entirely, you will not lose weight on The Three Rules. If you can, and you follow Rules 1 and 2, you will lose weight.

- **Do not eat potatoes in any form.**

Sweet Potatoes And Other Root Vegetables

The first question people ask me after I talk about potatoes is, "What about sweet potatoes?" We love sweet potatoes (sometimes called yams) too, but for whatever reason, we don't eat them nearly as often as white potatoes. We eat more now because people are realizing potatoes cause weight gain, so they are trying to get by with sweet potatoes. It doesn't work. Sweet potatoes are starchy, have a high glycemic index, and a high glycemic load. They are addictive, making the All or None approach best. They are against The Rules. Think of sweet potatoes as potatoes.

There are only a few other root vegetables that fall into the starchy category, but they are not as commonly eaten. Beets are on the list of many low-carb diets as food to be avoided. If they are canned or pickled, sugar is often added. If there is no sugar added, you can eat beets—they are not starchy enough to be a problem. No one got fat on beets. The key difference between beets and sweet potatoes is that there is far less starch in it. The glycemic load of beets is one-third that of sweet potatoes. Carrots are also sometimes on the "do not eat" lists. Forget it. Carrots have almost no carbs and very little sugar. Parsnips, turnips, and kohlrabi (which I do not recall ever eating) are other root vegetables of no concern. Rutabagas, yucca, and cassava are very starchy and to be avoided. Fortunately, that is easy to do.

- **Do not eat sweet potatoes**
- **The few other starchy root vegetables—rutabaga, yucca, and cassava are no good either.**

Corn

We talked about the products made from processed, refined corn, and those are definitely against The Rules. What about whole corn, either as sweet corn or as popcorn?

Sweet corn is against Rule 3. It is starchy and will raise your glucose if you eat enough. It would not raise your sugar as much as potato, gram for gram, but again, the All or None approach is best. I can easily go back for a second or third ear of corn, or another bowl of a sweet corn side dish. You don't want to eat anything in The Three Rules where moderation is critical. I don't pick out the few kernels of corn in a restaurant salad, but I would not order a side dish of corn.

Popcorn is really the only other unprocessed corn product to consider. It is starchy, but given the air in the popcorn, a serving size is rather low in carbohydrates. For that reason, many other carb-based diets will allow popcorn, <u>but I don't recommend it and consider it against The Rules</u>. It is addictive, will raise your glucose, and will interfere with your diet. When your glucose rises, the butter you put on the popcorn and the oil you used to make it will make the problem even worse. I find Rule 3 so very simple—No starchy fruits or vegetables, especially potatoes, corn, and rice. All corn is off limits under Rule 3.

- **Do not eat corn.**
- **Processed and refined corn products are especially against The Rules.**

Rice And Whole Grains

As I have mentioned, not every food or every food group is either great for the diet or bad for it, black or white. Grains are definitely the biggest gray area. Refined grains are part of Rule 2, and I also put grains in Rule 3, knowing that some readers will write me to tell me that grains are not fruits or vegetables. Fine, I accept it, but I think that is semantics. I don't care what you call them.

White rice and its products are definitely against Rule 2 because of refining and processing. Brown rice is a gray area food, because it has a moderate glycemic index and glycemic load. It has more digestible starch than oats, barley and most other grains. Therefore, its glycemic load is not that good. It is also very difficult to eat any rice in moderation. When you make it at home, you would have to be very careful not to overeat it. Since it has that potential, you are far better off not eating brown rice at all. Consider all rice to be against Rule 3.[23] It is not worth sacrificing your diet and weight for any form of rice.

There are some people who can eat brown rice without a problem. Some people will continue to lose weight, and when they reach their goal, they can eat brown rice and not gain their weight back. I am not such a person. If you want to try brown rice, be very careful. If your weight doesn't come off as expected, or if you start to gain your lost weight back, blame it on the brown rice and stop it. For most of us, Rule 3 works best—Do not eat starchy foods, especially potatoes, corn, and rice. I recommend that if you try eating brown rice, put additional wording into Rule 3 for yourself, something like "Do not eat starchy vegetables or fruits, especially potatoes, corn, and white rice—brown rice is fine." Call it a Rule 3 Variation. Maybe it will work for you, but you still need to have an ironclad Rule to follow. You don't want to accumulate little exceptions to the Rules. One of the most important parts of The Rules, remember, is that it is All or None. I don't eat brown rice, but your Rule Variation may work for you.

Other than rice, the other grains, if unprocessed, are acceptable. I discussed oats extensively with Rule 2—unprocessed oat groats and steel-cut oats have more resistant than digestible starches, and the glycemic index and load are low, so they are fine. Barley, quinoa, wheat berries, farro and nearly all other unprocessed, non-rice grains are fine. Virtually all wheat products are refined and processed and against Rule 2. Wheat berries, occasionally seen in health food stores, is the name for the groats of wheat—so they are unprocessed. Wheat berries are fine, but make sure you see the whole grain itself in the food, that it is not refined wheat or wheat berry flour.

Just avoid all rice, corn and processed wheat, which again is almost all the wheat you will see in food. If you come across a grain you don't know, search for its glycemic load. If it is similar to quinoa and barley, and it is unprocessed and unrefined, eat it if you want. Again, except for

---

[23] The Three Rules prohibits bad carbs. In most instances, that means that the glycemic index or load are high. Brown rice, along with a few other exceptions, has a moderate glycemic load, but since it is so difficult to eat in small amounts, like pasta, we eat far more carbs than the 50 grams of the glycemic index, ruining our diet. All rice is against The Rules.

rice, most unprocessed grains are fine in The Three Rules, but you cannot be ridiculous. Don't test The Rules by eating a pound of hulled barley at one sitting. You don't have to moderate or measure any of the acceptable grains, but don't be ridiculous.

I spent a lot of time talking about grains, probably more than was necessary. I don't want you to worry about it much. Our chief goal is weight loss and then weight control. Rule Three is straightforward. Avoiding potatoes, corn, rice, and a few other foods is all it takes to follow Rule 3.

- **Do not eat rice of any kind.**
- **Do not eat any ground or processed wheat.**
- **All other whole grains are fine, but don't be ridiculous.**

Bananas

Bananas and plantains are really the only fruits worth mentioning that have significant digestible starch. I sometimes say that no one got fat eating bananas. While that is almost certainly true, bananas have a lot of starch, so we need to talk about them. If you stick to the absolute Rules and the All or None approach, then don't eat bananas. Plantains and unripe bananas have starch that is fairly resistant, and the glycemic index is reasonably low. Ripe and overripe bananas have a higher glycemic index. I will eat bananas on the green side. If you think you want to do that, feel free. If you want to decide that bananas are not worth eating, don't eat them. I would not eat ripe or overripe bananas, but I have never seen people gain weight on bananas, and people just don't develop a habit of eating too many of them. If you eat a lot of them, try the less ripe ones. I may be drawing too thin a line of distinction, and I don't think your success will hinge on your decision about bananas regardless of the ripeness of bananas you enjoy. If you notice, the Rule reads "especially potatoes, corn, and rice," because they are the only starchy vegetables or fruits that we eat regularly enough to make much of a difference. If you eat lots of ripe bananas, cassava, yucca or a few other starchy things, you will have to make a change.

- **Be careful with ripe or overripe bananas**

Squash

There are many varieties of squash. The summer squashes are zucchini and the classic yellow squash. Winter squashes are acorn, butternut, pumpkin and related varieties. Summer squashes are less starchy than winter squashes, but even the winter squash has much less digestible starch than potatoes, sweet potatoes, corn, or rice. They have an appreciable amount of fiber, do not raise blood glucose much, and will not affect your weight loss plan. I don't consider them starchy vegetables. Eat squash, summer or winter, just don't add the brown sugar.

Starchy Food Additives

There are few foods prohibited by Rule 3, just potatoes, sweet potatoes, corn, rice, and a few others. You also need to avoid packaged and prepared foods that use the starch from fruit and vegetables, and you have to be careful in reading the labels. Even some replacement milks and yogurts have these additives. It is obvious when the ingredients list includes corn starch that you shouldn't eat it. Adding corn starch (or flour because of Rule 2) to a sauce is worse than eating the corn itself—it is concentrated starch. But what about tapioca or maltodextrin or other additives?

Tapioca is starch from cassava, which I briefly mentioned earlier. It is a common additive, especially to gluten-free products. Maltodextrin is a starch from corn. Don't eat either. Every once in a while, I read a label and there is something I never heard of; I look it up, and it is a starch. Look up words until you know the various names for food starches. This is just like Rule 1, where you have to learn the dozens of words for sugar. Fortunately, most of us have smartphones and internet access, and you can easily look a word up.

Remember, All or None is the best approach. Since there is no way to tell just how much corn starch is added when it is on the label, don't eat it at all. There are many other things to eat. The same holds true with restaurants or other settings when you do not make the food. I was at a party recently and was told there were no carbs in a dish. We were chatting, and I saw someone dumping corn starch into the sauce without measuring how much he was using. Would eating that have killed me? Of course not. But why ruin a diet with corn starch? I would rather have had an ear of corn or a Sourdough Jack Burger. So eat with intent; find out what is in the food you are eating. Don't eat starchy fruits or vegetables, and don't eat foods prepared with the starch from them.

Part 4: Common Questions and Misconceptions

Sometimes simple things appear complicated and vice versa.

Over the years, I have seen people fail, including myself, over minor errors or misunderstandings of The Rules. I will include some of these common mistakes and some tips I have that may help you succeed. I will repeat some pointers I have made earlier, because I feel they are important. It is a terrible feeling to fail at any diet or any plan over a simple misunderstanding. If you stray from the diet, make it count, enjoy it, then go right back to work. Don't ruin the plan over something simple.

How Strict Are The Rules?

To succeed at something important, it always takes hard work and discipline. If that is being strict, I accept it.

A theme throughout this book has been how very easy it is to gain weight and how difficult it is to lose it. You cannot lose weight without work. That is a simple, undeniable fact. Trying to find wiggle room to keep eating something you like rarely works. It is up to you to decide if it is worth the work required. Giving up some foods you like is a big deal. But there are still many wonderful foods to eat on the Three Rules. I do not eat tofu and broccoli all day long. I promise.

You may be lucky. You may find that you can follow The Rules 90% and still succeed. Most people cannot. I cannot. I have come to grips with the reality that I cannot go outside The Rules and keep my weight in control. Perhaps I could get away with one Sourdough Jack Burger a month, or one bagel and cream cheese every other Sunday. But I have failed many times trying things like that in the past. There may be recovering alcohol abusers who can have a drink the first day of every month. For every such person, I would bet there are a hundred who relapse after that one drink.

All Or None And All In

I have discussed the All or None philosophy of the Three Rules, probably more times than you want to hear. I believe that All or None is what makes this diet work for most people. There are other diets that cut back on bad carbs, but the failure rate of these diets is high, because you have to moderate your intake. That takes willpower. Eating one thin mint cookie, a few french fries, one Lindor chocolate truffle—that is difficult. Not having even a taste of something? That to me is easier. I take pride in it and have a sense of accomplishment. I feel the same way when I don't have a glass of wine. If I don't have one, I cannot have two and wake up with a headache. One treat often leads to two. Zero never leads to one and so two is impossible. People say that alcohol is not a fair comparison, that you don't have to drink, but you do have to eat. That is a fallacy. You do have to drink, but you do not have to drink alcohol. You do have to eat, but not sugar, processed carbs, or starchy fruit or vegetables.

I recommend The Three Rules every day. I saw 20 patients today, about 8 were here for routine visits, and I recommended The Three Rules about five times. Each time I recommend The Rules, I tell them not to start unless they are committed. You must be All In. I tell them to put all their effort into it. I only recommend All or None. You will succeed if you go All In and eat All or None. If you do not, you may fail. You will probably fail.

All or None refers to the fact that you can essentially eat all you want within the Rules, provided that you eat none of the food against the Rules. Yes, if you eat buckets of fruit at a time (see later in this section), then you could overwhelm your body's ability to handle the sugar and gain weight. But that scenario is so rare that I don't worry about it. Much more likely than eating buckets of fruit is eating a cookie or two, or a small bowl of ice cream. A cookie or a little ice cream is not *none*. That will ruin almost any diet. One sample at Costco leads to several; one ear of corn leads to two; one Hershey Kiss leads to a bowl.

I explained The Rules to a patient today. They said that they already are doing it because they don't eat much bread. Please do not think that way. Not eating much doesn't mean anything. First, who defines "much?" Second, as we have discussed, the human body is very good at storing fat from just a little extra energy. It does not take "much" bread or sugar to ruin your diet. None—that works. It is easier to follow, and it takes less willpower. If you asked an alcoholic you love if they drank today, you would never want the answer to be, "not much."

This diet is not for everyone, but it works if you do it. Do not start The Three Rules plan unless you are All In. If you want to succeed in anything, that is your best chance. Devote all your energy to the Three Rules, and you will succeed. That philosophy holds true in so many things—learning a language, succeeding in your job, doing well in school. If you focus, devote all your efforts to it, and go All In, you will succeed.

Can You Still Enjoy Eating?

Can you still enjoy eating? With near certainty, you will enjoy eating more. You will have to give up the immediate pleasure of rocky road ice cream, but you will gain the deeper pleasure of control over what you eat. How many times have you woken up regretting the amount of unhealthy food you ate the day before? Have you ever felt good about yourself after overeating fast food? Eating healthy is like exercise. You will nearly always feel good after having done it. Feeling good about yourself is the best enjoyment there is.

Sure, but will I enjoy eating? I know that is a different question. I only eat food I enjoy. I eat steak, ham, chicken, salmon, shrimp, pork roast, and all kinds of soups, all on a regular basis. I enjoy them all. We eat plenty of vegetables—roasted, steamed, sautéed, all with wonderful sauces. Apples, oranges, grapefruit and berries—cheeses, cold cuts, and eggs. I can go on and on.

My wife, who has not had a weight problem, enjoys our meals. (I do most of the cooking, and while it is possible that she is fibbing a bit, she has yet to kick me out of the kitchen.) When our son is home from college, he eats with us most nights and has never gone to McDonald's with his friends after an unfinished meal. In fact, his friends have told him that the dinners they have had at our house are some of the best meals they have had in a long time. Since I went All In on The Rules about six years ago, I have been essentially All or None. The rare times I went off the plan, I did it deliberately, with intent, for a 50-year anniversary party or some other special event. I have not woken up regretting what I ate the day before. Not a single time. That is a wonderful feeling. It makes me want to work hard that day and every day.

I want you to experience the same enjoyment. If you continue what you are doing now, or if you start The Rules or some other diet plan and fail because you were not strict enough, you will feel bad about yourself. Then you will definitely not enjoy eating; at least not for longer than a few minutes.

Cheat Days

Many diets allow or even recommend cheat days. This is when you "cheat" on your diet once a week, once a month, or whatever. Based on my All or None philosophy, you probably figured out that I am against cheat days. First, I don't like the word "cheat" in this situation. I am happy with The Three Rules; I am proud that I have been on it for several years; I am happy with the success it has brought me; and I am enjoying my life more. I would not be cheating the diet if I ate a Sourdough Jack Burger. I would be cheating myself, hurting myself.

Most of us will not stop at one cheat day a week or a month. It often leads to more and more straying from the diet. This is exactly why Alcoholics Anonymous does not recommend a cheat day of drinking, why no drug counselor recommends a cheat day for heroin, and no one recommends a cheat day in your marriage. I believe that we should decide how we want to live and stick with it the best we can. Do I ever eat anything off The Rules? It is rare, but it happens. But when I eat something against The Rules, I do it happily, with intent, not cheating anyone or anything. And then, immediately after, I am back with The Rules.

You Cannot Be Ridiculous

Human beings can gain weight without bad carbs. In fact, we could probably gain weight with no carbs. If you ate enough pure protein or good carbs, and you did it quickly enough, you might overwhelm your ability to control the glucose rise. You might gain weight. In my experience, this is very difficult and uncommon. Most people would fill up and stop eating before their glucose rose too high, since protein and fat suppress appetite. When people gain weight by gorging on food, it is almost always from carbs.

I tell people that they can eat what they want if it is not against The Rules. You do not need to measure foods or count carbs. You can eat three apples or a pound of shrimp. But if you go crazy, eating ridiculous amounts, say a 60 ounce steak or several pounds of shrimp dipped in butter, then I am not so sure you would still lose weight. Doing that is ridiculous. I also criticize myself when I "eat from the trough." By this I mean sitting next to a bowl or bag of food and eating from it all day long. That is not a recipe for success, though if the food is within The Rules, you might be okay. My point is this: eat what you want, but don't be ridiculous and don't eat from the trough.

What About Protein And Fat?

If you eat something without carbohydrates, did you really eat it?

The Three Rules affects only what you eat that has carbohydrates—sugar, processed and refined carbs, and starchy foods. Protein and fats have no sugar, no starch, and no carbs at all. If all you ate were protein and fats, you would lose weight, unless you went crazy and ate all day long. This is the basis of the ketogenic and Atkins diets. (As you recall, people do not stay on these diets and regain their weight quickly.)

Since we are not banning all carbohydrates, can you still eat all the protein and fat you want and lose weight? If you are strict with the Rules, you can. If you never stray from The Three Rules, then all protein and fat are neutral. They do not help, and they do not hurt. Since you give up bad carbs when obeying the Three Rules, you have to eat something else—protein, fat and good carbs are all you have to choose from. That is all there is. Fortunately, all three categories can be delicious.

If you don't follow The Rules closely, protein and fat will just add to your weight gain. A hamburger bun by itself, clearly against The Rules, is bad enough. If you put a double cheeseburger with mayo on it, you will definitely not lose weight, and the extra calories will cause you to gain weight. Calories from fat, protein, and carbs matter. They matter much, much more if you eat the bad carbs. If you don't eat the bun or anything else against The Rules, you will lose weight, even if you eat the double cheeseburger. There are a few other issues worth mentioning about protein and fat, but they are straightforward.

Meats And Fish

Since you will give up bad carbs, then you will eat good carbs, protein, and fat. Unless you are a vegan, much of the protein will be red meat, poultry, and fish, with some from nuts and vegetables. Vegans have to get all their protein from plants—more difficult, but still easily done. As

I just said, meats and fish, having no carbs, are always fine on The Three Rules. If you eat bad carbs, then you will gain weight from the protein and fat in anything you eat. If you don't eat bad carbs, you won't.

Be careful of a few things when eating meat and fish. Eating it at home is easy. Don't put anything on it that has sugar, processed and refined carbs, or starchy fruit and vegetables. When you eat out, or if you eat from a package, you have to watch out. If there is a label, read it. Beef jerky and cold cuts often have added sugar and starch, many sauces have outlawed foods in them, and most fried foods will have breading. If you are out, and there is no label, ask what is in it. If in doubt, don't eat it. Ask for sauce on the side, no sauce, or whatever you have to do. Don't let some breading on the chicken or sauce on your shrimp ruin your plans. Don't just eat it because it is there.

If it is your mother's fried chicken, and you want to eat it, that is up to you. But if you eat it, do so knowing that you are going against your plans, that it will affect your diet. Eat it with intent. Then start back with The Rules again, right after the meal.

Fats And Oils

Fats and oils are simple. If you only eat within The Rules, then they don't matter. If you eat bad carbs, then fats and oils make it worse. For health reasons, but not for weight loss, certain fats are better for you than others. Though there is some disagreement, olive and canola oil seem to be the best for heart health. I am still not sure about coconut oil, and most other plant derived oils are fine.

Meat and dairy fats may not be as good for you as plant oils, but they are not as harmful as previously thought. In fact, dairy fat, especially in yogurt and cheese, may lower the risk of cardiovascular disease and diabetes. Unless there is added sugar or other food additives made from starch, all dairy is within The Rules. Read the label and it is easy.

Eggs

Eggs have no carbohydrates, are an excellent source of protein, and fill us up for the day. Whole eggs or egg whites are the same for the purposes of The Three Rules. It should go without saying by now that you have to know what else is in the egg dish. Most omelets have no added sugar or processed and refined carbs, but ask or read the label of everything you eat. Clearly, if potatoes are in a side dish or in the egg dish itself, then it is against the Rules.

Unrelated to weight loss, the media and websites have droned on recently how eggs have no health risks. I believe that if a person has a low risk of coronary heart disease, then eating eggs in moderation has little risk. But, if someone has had a heart problem already, or if they are at especially high risk of a heart attack, they should talk to their doctor and probably cut back on eggs. Personally, I buy egg whites in cartons at Costco. It is inexpensive and simple to make into an omelet or scrambled egg dish. I will leave the issue of eggs and heart risk to you and your doctor, but as far as The Three Rules is concerned, eggs are good.

Special Topics

A few things need further explanation.

The media, the internet, and people you know cannot always be trusted. The problem is that much of what they say is true, but some is completely false. This is the case in every aspect of life, and diets are no exception. You will hear claims about what is missing from a diet like The Three Rules; unhealthy foods that should not be allowed; foods that The Rules allows that may raise blood sugar. There will be websites talking about a food additive that has one harm or another, and you will see ads and even medical sites claiming that some food or other will burn fat. I will explain a few of these special topics, but there is no reason for controversy. The Rules allow for a variety of approaches—you can follow the plan if you don't agree with some of my opinions about health, if are a vegan, if you keep kosher, if you only eat organic food, or if you have no dietary restrictions at all. Just don't eat foods against the Rules.

Remember that The Three Rules is designed to help you lose weight, not to solve every health problem. If there is a food within The Rules that you feel is harmful, don't eat it. If you are missing out on one or two otherwise healthy foods, try not to worry about it. The Three Rules allows for so much variety, this will not be an issue.

Is The Three Rules Diet Healthy?

We have discussed how The Three Rules will solve your weight problem. We know that bad carbs cause obesity and eliminating them results in weight loss. There are still some who believe that cutting carbs, even bad carbs, is unhealthy. I do not want to belabor the point—there are many, many studies showing the health benefits of eliminating sugar and refined carbohydrates. In fact, I was not going to even write this section, but a study came out this month confirming for the umpteenth time the cardiovascular benefits of cutting out bad carbs.[24] This study should put to rest any further concerns of a low glycemic index diet, and by extension, The Three Rules. Over twelve months, improving the diet with respect to sugar and refined carbohydrates improved blood pressure, body weight, waist circumference fasting glucose, hemoglobin a1c (a measure of overall glucose levels), triglycerides, and cholesterol.

We already know that losing weight helps all the medical problems associated with obesity. It is also clear that losing weight on The Three Rules, eliminating bad carbs, directly benefits the factors that contribute to cardiovascular disease. If anyone tries to say otherwise, this study and a simple internet search should be enough to satisfy them.

Aren't There Healthy Foods Against The Rules And Unhealthy Foods That Obey The Rules?

Most of the foods within The Rules are also good for us for reasons other than weight control. Fruits, vegetables, beans, nuts, dairy, lean meats, fish, and chicken are all healthy, and they are all fine on the Three Rules plan. Most of the foods against the Rules, such as pastries, other sweets, pasta, bread, and cereal are unhealthy or at least not especially good for us. There are exceptions. You will not eat a few otherwise healthy foods, such as brown rice and corn. I accept it. There will always be healthy foods you do not eat. There are hundreds of fruit and vegetables that you will not eat because they are unavailable where you live, or you don't like them. One trip down the aisle at an Indian market (one of my favorite places to shop), and you will realize you have never heard of most beans and vegetables that exist. You can never eat all the healthy foods. So if you miss out on a few because they are against the Rules, so be it. Overall, you will be much healthier having lost the weight.

I also want to make a comment about the word "healthy." Just yesterday, I mentioned to a diabetic patient that they should give up potatoes to help with weight loss and to lower their glucose readings. They said

---

[24] Martínez-González, M. A., et al (2019). Carbohydrate quality changes and concurrent changes in cardiovascular risk factors: a longitudinal analysis in the PREDIMED-Plus randomized trial. *The American Journal of Clinical Nutrition, 111*(2), 291–306. https://doi.org/10.1093/ajcn/nqz298

they thought potatoes are healthy. Healthy is an ambiguous term. Like most foods, potatoes have good and bad properties. If you are looking for tasty, inexpensive nutrition, it is great. The potato has been beneficial in the past when food was scarce. Potatoes have vitamins that we need to live. But if you have a weight problem, then potatoes are not healthy. Many foods are like that. Breakfast cereal has vitamins and fiber. It is only unhealthy if you want to lower your blood sugars and lose weight. Most things in life have upsides and downsides. A car is vital if you need to drive to work. Yet we all know that there are thousands of serious car accidents a year. Try to think about the benefits and negatives of all foods. Is eating a food outside The Rules, if it is healthy in some ways, worth the downsides? Is one health benefit worth the negative effect on your weight? Since obesity is one of the leading causes of morbidity and mortality, I would rather you lose the weight and find another way to get the health benefits from potatoes or any other food that is against The Rules.

Two analogies to giving up some healthy foods to lose weight are allergy and alcohol (again). Nuts are good for you, but if you are allergic, the health benefits of nuts are clearly outweighed by the negatives. Shell-fish, milk, and strawberries are healthy foods to which people are often allergic. You would never advise someone to eat them anyway. Alcohol likely has some health benefits, but an alcoholic is advised not to drink alcohol, regardless of the possible benefits. I think of bad carbs the same way. Sure, there are some benefits to a few foods that are against The Rules. Don't eat them—the downside is too great.

There are also some iffy or downright unhealthy foods that are within The Rules. Trans-fat, the worst food additive, which used to be in mar-garine and some shortening and is rarely seen at all anymore, is within the Rules, as are all fats. I don't recommend eating trans-fat. Processed red meat most likely has health risks. But this is a book about weight. I recommend to my patients to avoid trans-fat, minimize processed red meat, and overall, choose fish and poultry over unprocessed red meat, though red meat is likely nowhere near as bad as we thought in the past. Eating a lot of eggs if you have heart or other artery disease may not be a good idea. There are undoubtedly other unhealthy foods that are al-lowed in The Three Rules plan. I cannot cover every food. If you are concerned about food that might be bad for you, then don't eat it, or eat less of it. There are countless ways that we can be healthier. For most people, weight is the most important problem. Stick to The Three Rules, and you will solve that problem. After that, if you want to tackle other health issues, related to food or not, that is up to you, and I recommend it.

Are There Fat Burning Foods?

You have probably seen claims of a food "burning fat." There is no such thing. Eating any specific food never helps any diet—it is what you remove from your diet, what you no longer eat that matters. Eating an allowed food does not negate the prohibited food's effects. Fiber in the diet can blunt glucose rise and help some. Protein and fat in a meal can also lessen glucose rise of eating sugar. But eating protein, fat or fiber does not cause weight loss or fat-burning.

This morning, I was explaining Rule 2 to a patient, and they asked what I ate for dinner last night. I said I had sautéed shrimp and brussels sprouts. She told me she doesn't like brussels sprouts. Fine, there are many things I don't like to eat either. Eating brussels sprouts is not the important thing. Eating all the vegetables in the world doesn't help. But it doesn't hurt. So when you remove the fettuccine alfredo, you have to replace it with something. If you replace it with shrimp and brussels sprouts, or steak and a caesar salad, you are good. The important thing is that I did not have the pasta and dinner rolls. That is the crux of The Three Rules. Since I had to eat something, I chose shrimp and brussels sprouts, but there is a nearly infinite variety of foods I could have chosen. Nothing you choose will burn fat. It is the removal of junk food that burns the fat. You replace the junk food with whatever you want that is within the Three Rules.

Dried Fruit

The most popular dried fruit is raisins. Grapes have some sugar in it, of course, but they are not a problem on The Three Rules. It takes a lot of grapes to raise your sugar, so the glycemic load is reasonably low. We just rarely eat massive amounts of grapes at a sitting. Raisins do have the issue of allowing us to eat much more at a sitting. But I don't worry about it. No one gets fat on raisins. They just don't raise our blood glucose to the level that added sugar or the other prohibited foods do.

Prunes, apricots, figs, dates, cranberries, cherries, and mangoes are other commonly encountered dried fruit. Similar to raisins, they usually are not a problem. If you eat any of these foods to excess, you will probably encounter some level of gastrointestinal disturbance before the sugar becomes a problem. I have not seen dried fruit interfere with anyone's weight loss. If you ate 5 or 6 servings in a sitting, I suppose it could, but I doubt that will be an issue for you. I have mentioned that some borderline foods, such as brown rice, are prohibited, because they are addictive. If you are a dried mango addict, then you are probably the only one. I would then consider not eating it. Otherwise, no one got fat on dried mangoes.

Remember, I am assuming you are reading the labels and paying attention to Rule 1. Many dried fruits, especially cranberries, blueberries, cherries, and mangoes have added sugar. Read every single label of everything you eat. Do you want to ruin your diet plans on dried mangoes because there is added sugar? You could have eaten a fresh mango, an apple, or anything else. Dried fruits are fine. Dried fruits with added sugar are not.

Artificial Sweeteners

We know that sugar-sweetened food is harmful, causing weight gain, diabetes, and a host of other obesity related problems. Sugar has been linked to cancers, heart disease and other disorders not necessarily related to weight. We act as if we are addicted to sugar. But what about artificial sweeteners?

Artificial, also called non-nutritive, sweeteners have zero sugar, zero carbs, and usually zero or negligible calories. Aspartame, in Equal and NutraSweet, sucralose, in Splenda, and stevia, in Truvia and others, are the most popular. Some are natural, others not, but that doesn't make them good. Tobacco is natural, and so is sugar.

We consume the most artificial sweeteners in our diet drinks, especially diet sodas, and some people drink quite a bit of it. When I was in medical school, my roommate and I went through so much Diet Coke, it was embarrassing. Even now, I occasionally go on a binge of diet soda, drinking several a day for weeks. Then I realize what I am doing and stop for a while. As with many things we like, we can become addicted.

Are the sweeteners bad for us? That depends on what you mean, but they do not cause weight gain and do not interfere with weight loss. Anytime you study something and look for a harmful effect, you are likely to find it. High doses of some of these products, in animals at least, can cause problems. Sucralose has been linked to some gastrointestinal illnesses, and some people get migraines and other issues with aspartame. In general, though, they are well tolerated and safe. There are experts who believe that using artificial sweeteners increases appetite. That may be true, but with The Three Rules, that is not much of an issue. I notice that when I don't use any sweeteners, other foods taste sweeter and better.

There is another group of low-calorie ingredients called the sugar alcohols. They include erythritol, maltitol, xylitol and a few other "ols." They are in low-sugar food products such as protein bars. They are not quite zero calories, but we can consider them to be sugar free and essentially zero carb. They are fine on the Three Rules plan, but in excess, all sugar alcohols except erythritol can cause diarrhea and bloating. I avoid them because I am susceptible to this side effect, but you are free to try them.

I tell my patients that there may be an occasional problem with artificial sweeteners, but nowhere near the problems caused by sugar. If your choice is regular soda or diet soda, drink diet soda. If your choice is diet soda or water, tea, or coffee, drink the water, tea or coffee. All sugar-free sweeteners are fine on the Three Rules plan and should not interfere with losing weight or keeping it off. I try not to use them much, because I develop a habit, as I do with many things. And even though they are generally safe, I don't like the idea of eating anything that is not definitely good for me, especially if it is hard for me to quit.

A Few More Words About Food Additives

I have said many times that if you are going to break The Rules, then do it with intent, and make it count. Nowhere is it more important than with food additives. To fail in your diet due to a food additive that you don't even taste is a shame. Sweeteners from the list of about 60 different names for sugar are easy to spot. If you aren't sure, look it up.

In the chapter on Rule 3, we talked about various starchy food additives. Some of these have chemical sounding names, such as maltodextrin. It is added to a lot of mixes and bars, and it is converted to glucose easily. Avoid it completely. Various starches are often added to change subtly the taste of food and to thicken it. These are common in low-fat foods, replacing the fat's effect on food texture. When the word starch is on the label, don't eat it. You might see corn starch, tapioca starch, or modified food starch.

Thickening sauces within The Rules can be a challenge. You can try various gums, such as guar gum and xanthan gum. If you use them at home, read instructions on the internet, because you do not use them as you would flour or cornstarch. Be aware that a thickened sauce at a restaurant usually has flour or cornstarch in it.

Carrageenan, made from seaweed, is a food additive that is making the rounds on the internet. It is put into a lot of beverages, such as soy and almond milk. It has no carbs and no calories and will not affect your diet. You don't taste it, so there is no risk of becoming addicted to it. Some but not all studies suggest there may be health risks consuming it in large amounts for extended periods. For the purposes of The Rules, carrageenan is fine. If you believe the negative stories, avoid it if you want.

There are far too many food additives to name them all. New ones and alternative names for old ones appear regularly. I look them all up. Even with the internet, it is not always easy to determine if a specific additive is against The Rules. If there are no carbs at all, then it is definitely fine. If there are no calories, then you know there are no carbs, and it is fine. If there are carbs, and it is another name for sugar, don't eat it; if not, look up the glycemic index. If the index is lower than about 20, it is probably fine. I am not saying that the additive is good for you, but it is unlikely to ruin your diet. Don't ruin your diet for something you don't even taste. Again, eat with intent. If you go off the Three Rules, make it count.

A Few Other Issues

Not everything is about the actual eating. You can Help yourself in other ways.

We have discussed all you need to know about eating within The Three Rules. All the rest is follow-through. There are a few things not directly related to eating that will help you succeed: Exercise, cooking, and shopping.

What About Exercise?

I talked about exercise earlier. It is such an important topic and so often misunderstood that I want to go into more detail. Exercise is unnecessary with the Three Rules. Exercise does not prevent weight gain if you don't eat right. Patients tell me all the time that they gained 20 or more pounds because something interfered with their activity level or their ability to exercise. It is winter, their job is now more sedentary, they had more family stress, or they suffered an injury. It is rarely if ever the genuine cause of the weight gain. Few people gain weight, regardless of activity level or exercise, without eating too much of the wrong foods. Fortunately, you can lose weight and keep it off despite not exercising.

Does exercise help with weight loss? Of course it does, but as we discussed, not much unless you change your diet. It helps weight loss by blunting any glucose rise in the blood, making fat storage less efficient. And exercise burns fat. Aerobic exercise also helps lower the risk of many medical problems, especially cardiovascular disease. Over the last several years, strength training, such as weightlifting, has been shown to have additional health benefits. Almost everything tested improves with strength training: increased muscle mass, fat loss, diabetes, cholesterol levels, cardiovascular disease, stroke risk, bone strength, depression, and even overall mortality. Low muscle strength is an independent predictor of premature death, seen in this study and many others.[25] I recommend that nearly everyone engage in both aerobic exercise and strength training.

For overall health, I try to exercise every day, with strength training three days a week. Since I follow The Rules, I do not need the exercise to keep my weight off—I do it for all the other benefits. I have to eat more when I exercise, just to avoid losing too much weight. When I exercise more than typical, say on a hiking trip to Glacier National Park, I have to eat a great deal more, or I come home several pounds low. I usually eat much more dried fruit, whole grains, and nuts when exercising that much. Remember, it is not impossible to gain weight on The Rules, but it is difficult. But that doesn't mean that you will gain weight if you don't exercise. Just stay strict to The Rules.

I recommend you exercise. I recommend you do it every day if possible, but at least 3-4 days per week. It helps with overall health and weight management, as I have said, but more importantly, it helps you make the right food choices. When we exercise, we feel better, both physically and about ourselves. We have a sense of accomplishment. That leads to good, healthy choices. After 45 minutes on a treadmill, or lifting weights, I would not consider eating junk food and ruining it. Skipping planned exercise, for whatever reason, can lead to the attitude, "Screw it. I didn't exercise, I might as well give up on the entire day and eat at McDonald's." I have done it myself so many times I cannot tell you.

When patients explain their 20 pound weight gain by their lack of exercise, there are two points I try to mention tactfully. First, you don't gain 20 pounds by lack of exercise alone. It takes a change in eating habits. Some people honestly believe that their diet hasn't changed. But it can be subtle: a few more restaurant meals or takeout; an extra dessert at night; two more beers in the evening. Regardless, if you eat right, on The Three Rules, you will not gain weight, whether or not you exercise.

But the other point I make is more important. You can almost always find a way to exercise and stay active, regardless of what is happening in

[25] Ortega, F. B., et al (2012). Muscular strength in male adolescents and premature death: cohort study of one million participants. *BMJ*, *345*(nov20 3), e7279. https://doi.org/10.1136/bmj.e7279

life. Of course, a true family crisis takes precedence over exercise. But otherwise, you can usually find time to go for a walk outside, go up and down stairs at the library, march in place for 20 minutes watching television, walk the mall if the weather is bad, or go to the gym, if you can afford a membership. Even a broken leg will not stop you, if you are motivated. You can do upper body exercise by push-ups against the sofa, light weights over and over, pulling up from the chair, or if allowed, walking with crutches—which is far more exercise than walking without a broken leg. It is difficult exercising with an injury, or marching in place for 20 minutes when the weather is bad outside, but who said life was easy? In the beginning of the book, I said losing weight is hard. Exercise is hard too. Do it anyway.

How To Cook

Obviously there is no way I can teach you to cook in a few paragraphs. I cook most days, but it would be a stretch to say that I am a talented cook. Fortunately, you do not need to be one to make healthy, tasty meals that follow The Three Rules. I expect you do not need any advice on preparing most breakfasts and lunches. Scrambled eggs, yogurt and fruit, a cheese plate, vegetables and peanut butter, tuna salad—I think you can manage.

What about dinners, the meal most of us look forward to? I would divide dinners into two categories: casual and formal. Most of the weekday meals would be casual. A more formal meal would be on the weekends, and the truly formal meal would be parties or holidays.

I know that what I am writing here does not apply to many or most of you, because it is likely that you have more cooking skill and more imagination than I do. If you skip the rest of this section, I promise that I am fine with it. Most of the casual meals would center on a protein, like steak, chicken, fish or vegetarian proteins like beans. A side of vegetables or a salad would be common. Look for recipes online or in books on how to prepare them the way you like them. Many websites let you search "low carb." I assume you know the sites or can find them, but I use Epicurious.com, Food.com, and Allrecipes.com the most. For a subscription, cooksillustrated.com is superb, and I have learned some of my favorite recipes from them. Many of the low-carb recipes do not completely adhere to The Three Rules. That is fine, since it is simple, with a few tweaks, to make the meal fit The Rules. If there is added sugar, use sucralose, stevia, or aspartame, calculating the amount based on the recommendations on the sweetener labels. If there is a thickener such as corn starch or flour, then either leave it unthickened, or thicken it with xanthan gum, guar gum, flaxseed, or a few other products you can find online. Read the instructions since I have ruined a dish or two with some of these thickeners. To thicken a soup, you can use also puréed lentils or mung beans.

A formal meal is not really that different. I spend more time making it perfect, and if I have altered the recipe significantly, I try it out before I serve it to others. When we have a big party, with multiple courses, we may make some dishes that are against The Rules. You don't have to eat it, just as some vegans serve meat to guests and do not eat it themselves. If you feel that the sweet potato casserole will tempt you on Thanksgiving, then just don't make it. Some people have no trouble eating whatever they want on a holiday, going right back to their diet plan the next day. I cannot always do that, so I just don't eat against The Rules. There is always, always more than enough to eat at a holiday dinner that is within The Rules.

Many of you may have a family member who will not be on your diet plan. Our son, when home from college, will often eat junk food and bad carbs. That is up to him. When he eats with us, he generally eats what we do. Sometimes, if he has a friend over, I make a separate side dish, like a rice pilaf—I know I can avoid eating rice. When he was in high school, I sometimes just made a separate meal for him. It was more work, but it was worth it not to eat the spaghetti marinara he wanted for dinner.

Ideally, everyone in your household would eat as you want to eat, but I know that is not always practical. I frequently hear from someone who fails at this diet because their spouse is an outstanding cook and makes food that is against The Rules. She might be a baker and makes the best bread. You will have to decide how important your weight is to you. I believe it is the most important health concern in non-smokers. So I decided that I will do what I think is best, regardless. You can always tell the baker in the family that you appreciate it, but you don't want to eat it. My alcohol analogy applies here as well. I often get gifts of wine from connoisseurs. I politely tell them I do not drink. I am sure that vegans do the same when their loved ones want to make them a prime rib for their birthday.

How To Shop

The vast majority of all foods are healthy and good for our weight. We often purchase the few bad ones. After describing The Rules and the general diet plan, I am frequently asked, "What do you eat?" The better question is really, "What do you buy?" We eat what we have at home, order at a restaurant, buy on a whim at a gas station or other store, and given to us for free—such as samples at a store, food at a party, or treats at the office. Free bad carbs can be handled quite easily by a tactful reply to the giver and an All or None approach. I will touch on this topic later.

When you are buying the food yourself, then you have an advantage. You have two steps to avoid breaking a Rule: don't buy it and then don't eat it. We all know that once you buy it, even if you tell yourself it is for a special occasion or it is for your child or spouse, you are likely to eat it. If it is in the house, you have to have willpower all the time. This is why someone who wants to quit smoking should never buy cigarettes and never keep them in the house, and why people with an alcohol problem should not have alcohol in the house. If a temptation is right in front of you for hours a day, you have to have discipline hours each day. I rarely keep bad carbs in the house, so I only really need willpower at the store. The rare times I have junk food in the house—like when my wife and son make Christmas treats—I have to be careful. I try to never have junk food in the house. I never buy it.

What do you do if you live with others who do not want to stick to The Three Rules? You have a few options. Ideally, you would convince them of the value of The Rules. This works best if you have a spouse or partner who also has a weight issue. Then you both want to avoid keeping bad carbs in the home. If you have a child, well, you are the boss, and you can make your own rules. If none of that is feasible, then you may have to buy the food they want. Some people, once they are following

The Three Rules for a while, can see bad carbs around the house and just not eat it. For most people, myself included until recently, it is just too difficult to avoid eating junk food that is around them. You can make a deal with your spouse, child, or roommate. Have an area of the pantry or refrigerator that is off limits to you. You can even lock it up. Putting a lock on a drawer or cabinet is not that difficult. It seems drastic, but if it helps you conquer your weight problem, then do it. Some parents lock their liquor cabinets, so this is not all that unusual.

Do not cave in and buy junk food at the store on a whim. The best prevention is a list—always go in with a list. That gives you a failsafe to keep you following The Rules: Don't put junk food on the list and don't buy anything not on the list. Then you won't have it in the house, and you won't eat it. Easy.

At the store, you will spend most of your time in the produce aisle, the meat and seafood area, and the dairy aisle. You may stop at a few other sections to get frozen fruit or vegetables, condiments, and so on. Don't even go in the bakery, the prepared foods section, the cereal aisle, or the candy aisle. Avoid the snack aisle unless you have nuts on your list. (The best place to buy nuts in my opinion is Costco—the highest quality and the lowest prices.) Stay away as much as possible from the parts of the store with foods that are against The Rules. Be careful at the ends of the aisles and at check-out, where they sell the especially tempting junk food.

Before buying food that has a label, read the ingredients. Repeating myself again, it is not grams of carbs or grams of sugar in the section called "Nutrition Facts" that is important. I look at this area because they often write about added sugars, which should be zero. They also list protein and fiber in the nutrition area. But it is the added sugar, which is always listed in the ingredients, that matters—remember that there are multiple names for sugars and refined carbs. I know I often mention reading the label. It is critically important. Don't buy anything without reading the label.

Part 5: Keeping It Off Forever

Losing weight and gaining it back is demoralizing. Don't let it happen.

I would be surprised if you have never lost weight and regained it. I have already told you how I have done it repeatedly. You may have heard of studies showing how this "yo-yo" of weight has health risks. That is not the biggest problem. It is demoralizing. We regret the weight gain and call ourselves stupid and weak. Feeling ashamed can then lead to more unhealthy choices. It can even make it more difficult to start another diet because we think we will just regain the weight again. If you look back to when the weight started returning, it is usually just a few days of poor food choices and lack of attention. It is rarely, if ever, that we say, "I want to just eat what I want, and I don't care if I regain the weight."

The Three Rules To Lose Weight And Keep It Off Forever is just what it says. The Rules plan works forever. There is not much difference in eating when you are losing weight and when you are keeping it off—you eat the same way. There is no transition from losing weight to keeping it off. In fact, I tell patients starting out on The Three Rules that you don't need a target weight or a goal amount of weight to lose, because losing weight and keeping it off are the same. You will lose the excess weight and just stay there.

For most people, there is nothing more to do once you lose the weight—just keep following The Rules. A few people will start to lose too much weight. This uncommon problem is easily managed, and we will talk about it later on. Generally, to keep the weight off, you just keep doing what you are doing. Your weight will remain stable.

As this part of the book will describe, the main difficulty in keeping weight off is that you have to stay focused. For the rest of your life, you will be tempted to break The Rules. Intentionally or not, people will encourage you to break them. You will have good days and difficult days and think of going back to old habits. I will go over some ways to avoid slipping. Remember what I have said—losing weight is hard. Keeping weight off forever is also hard. Do it anyway.

Losing Weight vs. Keeping It Off

When you follow the Three Rules, you will lose excess fat. You will naturally stay at the new weight.

Until the recent boom in the wealth and security of the Western world, we all ate mostly within the Three Rules. We ate little sugar or refined carbs, and when we ate starchy vegetables, it was not in the quantities we do now. Junk food was difficult to find. There was no fast food, takeout, pizza delivery and so on. When we ate bad carbs, the amount of exercise we did overwhelmed it. So we rarely needed to lose weight, and when we did, our work and our diet kept us from gaining it back. Now, we have to work hard to maintain our healthy weight. Fortunately, we will maintain our weight if we just continue to follow The Rules.

Should I Change The Rules?

You or someone you care about wants to and needs to lose weight. Start following The Three Rules right now. If you follow through on this commitment, then you are set for life. Just follow through. There are special challenges when you have lost the excess weight (fat, not muscle) and you are trying to keep it off. In theory, it is simple. Keep doing what you have been doing. Follow The Rules. There are times, though, when you want to or need to change The Rules, but do it with intent.

Why would you want to change The Rules, if you are doing well? You should not consider a major change—the risk of relapse is too great. There are only two times to even consider modifying The Rules, even in a small way. The first reason is risky—you may want to try a prohibited food again. The second is if you are losing too much weight. This is not common, and I will deal with it soon.

I do not recommend trying a prohibited food just because you miss eating it. I am too much of an addict to certain things, so I never do it myself. You may not be so addicted, so you may consider making a minor change, what I call a Rule Variation. You may allow corn, or sweet potato, or white rice, all prohibited by Rule 3. You might be tempted to try eating one candy bar a week. Again, it is very risky. If you do it, start very small, and do not give up the benefit of having a strict Rule to follow, so make a Rule Variation. Say to yourself that Rule 3 is now, "Do not eat starchy vegetables or fruits, except rice or sweet potatoes, or whatever." If you risk a candy bar a week, change Rule 1 to "Don't eat any food with added sugar except one Snickers bar on Sunday." That way there is a strict Rule again, and you can be accountable to it. Vague rules inevitably lead to failure. Do not wing it by saying to yourself that you partly obey Rule 3. Make your own new Rule 3, with the Variation. If you try something so risky, then I would strongly urge you to weigh yourself every few days. If you gain weight, then go back to the absolute strictest you can be with the Three Rules, without the Variation.

There are many other Variations of The Rules that my patients have created. Some add a processed and refined carbohydrate food weekly or even daily, others add rice or potatoes. A few people succeed, but most fail, allowing more and more prohibited food to creep back into their diet. It is up to you, but please be careful. The foods you add back are usually not worth the downside of gaining your weight back. I cannot stress enough that if you tweak a Rule, keep a strict Rule with the Variation, with wording that now includes your added foods.

Focus Every Day

We do many positive things every day, even when we are unhealthy in others. Most of us brush our teeth, take a shower, kiss our loved ones, tuck our kids into bed. Yet, attention to our diet is somehow not worth doing every day. Most people rate the health of themselves and their family as one of their top priorities. Yet, we don't act as if we truly believe it, and unless you smoke, what you eat is the most important thing for your health.

If you follow The Rules, you will succeed. Do it every day. Focus every day. Focusing on my diet helps me focus on everything else in my life. In the past, when I would lose focus and gain my weight back, I also lost focus on other important things. I might stop exercising, drink more alcohol, and mindlessly flip channels on television. Of course, we should have leisure time, relaxation, vacations, and so on. But think about it—do you stop brushing your teeth and showering on a vacation? If you want to succeed in anything, you have to focus. This is especially true with addictive things, like sugar and other bad carbs.

There are many reasons we lose focus on our diet. I have mentioned some already—injury, illness, job stress, holidays, a busy time in our lives, and occasionally serious crises. Sometimes we allow a friend to talk us into eating an addicting snack or dessert. We may feel bad saying no to office colleagues bearing treats. Whatever it is, we all are prone to losing concentration and diverting our attention from something important, like our health. We are not perfect. Don't waste energy on guilt or self-recrimination. If you do lose focus, and it likely will happen, recognize it and start immediately back with The Rules. If you slip up with any important goal in life, don't wait. Don't put it off until tomorrow or next week. You can regain focus immediately, the same day, or even the same moment that you lose it.

What If I Lose Too Much?

It may seem difficult to believe, but The Rules are so effective that some people continue to lose weight after they reach their goal. Sometimes they set their target weight too high, not realizing that with The Three Rules their weight will continue to come off. Sometimes they set a reasonable goal, and they continue to lose weight, becoming too thin. This has happened to me. You may think it is a good problem to have—I would indeed rather be losing too much weight (without illness) than be gaining too much weight. There are risks, though. It is tempting, in this situation, to just start eating bad carbs, perhaps potatoes one meal, or a dessert the next. Just like a treat day, or going off The Rules when you are upset or too busy to cook, it often leads quickly to gaining the weight back.

If you are losing too much weight, I recommend two things. First, find something within The Rules that you like, in my case, it is nuts. Eat more of them. I eat about a cup and a half of nuts a day. I roast raw almonds and walnuts and eat them morning and evening. That is over

1000 calories of nuts a day. Since I am 5 foot 5 inches, that is a lot of calories, more than any dietician in the past would recommend for weight management, given that I eat three meals a day in addition. Adding a lot more whole grains such as barley or quinoa can also stop unwanted weight loss.

If you prefer fruit to nuts, fine, eat much more fruit than you were eating while you were losing weight. Bananas, being a borderline fruit, would be an excellent choice, as would grapes, fine overall in the Rules, but relatively high in sugar. Eating a lot of grapes might overwhelm your system and cause some weight gain or at least minimize unwanted weight loss. You could also purposely eat two portions of whatever protein you eat for dinner, extra servings of vegetables, more cheese, it doesn't matter. If you eat an enormous amount of anything, even within The Rules, you are likely to stop losing weight. I have mentioned earlier that it is possible to fail to lose weight or even to gain weight within The Rules, but it is difficult. The Three Rules will not necessarily work if you do something crazy or ridiculous. If you do what I just recommended, while not crazy or ridiculous, it might stop you from losing too much weight. Monitor your weight, and when you stop losing, simply cut back. It should be easy to cut back on the foods you just added, unless you started eating something addictive, like ice cream.

It is rare that doing this will not stop your weight loss, but if you continue to lose weight, or if you just cannot eat more of any foods within The Rules, then you can try adding something against The Rules, making a Rule Variation, like we discussed earlier. Try to use something not typically that addictive, like rice, corn, or sweet potato. I don't recommend you eat potatoes because they are very addictive. The same holds for candy, pastries, or bread rolls. They are just too addictive, and like a cheat day, you are risking regaining all your weight back.

Whatever you do, I strongly recommend naming it a Rule Variation. That way you maintain the benefit of All or None. You still follow The Rules, you just tweaked one of them. Then, as in the earlier section, you can say to yourself for Rule 3, "Do not eat starchy vegetables or fruit— but I will eat sweet potatoes every other day." Or "Do not eat any food with processed… except one dinner roll every day." You get the idea. Make a Rule Variation and stick to it.

I generally recommend not weighing yourself that often. However, if you make a Rule Variation, I would weigh yourself at least weekly. When you stop losing weight, back off on what you have added to your diet. If you see a continued trend toward weight gain, then I would eliminate the Variation completely and go back to the strict Rules. I do not have an exact recommendation on the amount of weight gain, but I would not wait too long. If you had lost a few pounds more than you think you should have, I would stop the Variation when you gain that back. You may have to try different Variations in different amounts until you find the right balance.

I would not spend too much time on this issue, since it is not common at all. In most people, sticking to The Rules is all you need to do. You are not likely to lose more than you want. If it happens, as long as you pay close attention to what you are doing, there is little risk of making a minor Variation to The Rules. But don't lose focus. If you make a tweak, and you don't weigh yourself, you are likely to put it out of your mind. You may regain your weight and be right back where you started. I have seen it many times.

Part 6: Tips and Traps or How to
Live On The Three Rules

Success does not come from never making mistakes but in
never making the same one a second time.
George Bernard Shaw

Here is a grab bag of lessons I have learned over the years. Most of these pearls of wisdom came from my own mistakes and failures. I have already mentioned some tips earlier in various parts of the book, but I hope you will at least briefly read and think about them again. To work this hard and fail because of something avoidable is frustrating. We all make plenty of mistakes. Learning from someone else's is nice once in a while.

I could not group each tip or pitfall in a perfectly sensible way. I will simply go from one to the next. Many will be more important later in your plan, when you have lost the weight and are keeping it off, but it can help to at least read about them now so you can be ready for everything.

All Or None

For the last time, I promise, All or None is critically important. You are either following The Three Rules or you are not. You will succeed if you are All In. You may fail if you are not All In. Most experts believe this is the best approach with any addiction or recurring problem, such as alcohol, drugs, or gambling. Bad carbs, especially sugars, are similarly addictive. An alcoholic cannot get into trouble with alcohol if they do not have the first drink. No one can get into trouble with bad carbs, if they do not have the first bite.

Changing The Rules

You may be tempted to change The Rules, either on your own, or with one of the Variations I mentioned. That is your choice, but I have one recommendation, if you do so. Wait until you master The Rules first. Like any new endeavor, you want to have success with the strict rules before you make changes. When we have new staff in our office, we want to make sure they know the way to do things correctly first. Then they can fine-tune their work, cutting a small corner or two, and still be successful. If you bend The Rules from the start, and you fail, you cannot determine the cause of the failure. I strongly recommend you follow The Rules to the letter. Then, after you have success, if you feel the need to bend a Rule, start with small steps, making a Rule Variation, and paying close attention to your weight, so you can go back to The Rules strictly, and lose the weight again right away.

Eat With Intent

Every time you eat something, think to yourself whether you want to eat it. Eat with intent. We will be better off if we always act with intent. There would be far fewer accidents, fights, and obesity if we did. Just the simple act of thinking, "Do I want to eat this?" will usually keep us from eating it.

If you decide to break a Rule, do it with intent. You are less likely to regret it, and regret leads to further failures. If you mindlessly eat a bag of powdered donuts, you will regret it. If you feel it is the right thing to eat a Krispy Kreme chocolate glazed, then do it, do it with intent, and go right back to The Rules. Then you will succeed. You will lose weight, just not that day.

Make Your Own Meals

Make your own meals.[26] I know I am repeating myself, but it is important for The Three Rules, for health in general, and for many other reasons. When you buy the food and you prepare it, you can easily know that every single thing you eat and drink is within The Rules. You have an infinite number of options. There is no excuse for eating bad carbs if you make the food. It is that simple.

The idea that healthy food is expensive is simply not true. Chicken, fish, beef, pork, and shellfish are all reasonably priced now. I mention Costco's prices because that is where I shop, but low prices are available at many stores. Two whole chickens for ten dollars, salmon at $7.99 a pound, various cuts of meat at $3.99 a pound, and so on. I bought a 5 pound leg of lamb for $5.99 a pound and a wonderful bone-in ham for $2.99 a pound for Christmas dinner this year. It served ten of us, and we had a ton and a half of leftovers. I also made a bean dish—it was nearly free. The biggest meal of the year, for ten people, with leftovers, was about $60. The average dinner at my house is well under $10 and many are under $5.

Books have been written on the value of sitting down to a family dinner. The more we eat and socialize with our loved ones, the better. Takeout and restaurants rarely lead to the meaningful conversations that strengthen relationships.

Preparing a meal is only a chore if you decide it is a chore. I plan meals for the week and usually shop just once. Most of the weekday meals are simple, but on weekends, I try to make more elaborate dinners. Sometimes they are not so good. So what? That is how we learn. Cooking for yourself gives you a sense of accomplishment and can be a joy in and of itself. My wife just made pajamas for our son. I know many people who knit for fun, giving gifts to grandchildren or to charity. Knitting and sewing may have been considered chores at one time, but now we do it for

---

[26] As of this writing, we are in a shelter-in-place order in Minnesota. People are actually gaining weight. Even though restaurants are closed, people are not making their own meals—they are taking out prepared meals from restaurants and grocery stores. Before the lockdown, the title of this section was called, "Eat At Home." I changed it to remind us that eating at home used to mean "make your own meals."

fun and as an act of kindness. Cooking is the same thing, though I am the first to admit that my usual meal is not in the same league as my son's pajamas or the lap blanket I recently received from a patient. Embrace cooking as a fun, relaxing activity that saves money and helps you become healthy.

Do Not Keep Junk Food At Home

If you are at a restaurant, to avoid bad carbs you must have willpower for about an hour. If you go into a gas station, you have to be disciplined for a few minutes. If you are at home, and you have junk food there, you must be perfect continuously. Anything can slip you up. You are hungry and see the Oreo cookies. There is a problem at work that you are worried about, so you say that you will have one Dove chocolate bar. You allow yourself one bagel because your sister is staying with you. There is no limit to the excuses we make, allowing ourselves to stray from our plan. If the food is not in your home, you will not eat it in the home. It is that simple. Why set yourself up for failure? If a reformed alcoholic keeps alcohol in their home, they are at higher risk of relapse than if they do not have it in the home.

We live in the actual world. Many or most of us live with other people, and they may not have the same ideas as you do. They may want to keep bad carbs in the house. This can be managed, but it takes some work. The options are simple:

- You can insist that the food not be in the home. This requires a frank discussion, and depending on the relationship, it may be impossible.
- You can make keep the food in an area that you do not enter, like a certain closet or small refrigerator.
- You can even put bad carbs under lock and key. This is done commonly with alcohol.

Until it becomes a habit to follow The Rules, and you can avoid eating it even if the junk food is within reach, strongly consider keeping no bad carbs in the home. I had to do it 100% when I started. Now I still keep a junk food-free home, with only rare exceptions, mainly during the holidays when our son is at home.

These measures seem drastic, but being obese requires drastic measures. People with asthma do not allow smoking in their house. Those with newborns don't allow sick people to visit. Pregnant women do not drink alcohol at all. And obese people or those with an addiction to bad carbs don't allow junk food in the home.

Fat-Burning Foods

We discussed this before, and it is worth repeating. There are no fat-burning foods. There are no foods you can eat that will cause weight loss. A few foods may help you lose weight indirectly. Eggs and other proteins eaten early in the day may suppress appetite later. Cinnamon and perhaps some high-fiber foods may lower the glycemic index in a meal. But there are no foods that cause weight loss themselves. The key to The Three Rules is *removing* bad carbs (junk food) from your diet. Remove it entirely. Then, since you have to and should eat something, you eat foods within The Rules. The steak and green beans are not burning fat, but they are not offsetting the fat-burning you are getting from giving up the junk food.

Give up the junk food. Eat what is in The Rules. Try to ignore what you read and hear about fat-burning foods. Don't pay attention to get-thin-quick supplements or schemes. Even if they work, and they usually don't, you will not keep the weight off. You will learn nothing from it. You will not have the sense of accomplishment that comes with doing something yourself.

The Goal Should Be Absolute Adherence To The Rules

I cannot stress this enough. The Rules work if you stick to them. All or None works. Less than All or None may not and usually does not work. Do not expect this to be simple all the time. Every failure of The Rules plan or any diet happens when there is not strict adherence. In a low-calorie diet, if you have a few hundred extra calories here or there, you will probably fail. If you are on Weight Watchers, eat a few extra points, and you will fail. I ask patients what they are doing to lose weight, and they often say, "I am kind of doing South Beach" or "sort of counting calories." They are rarely successful.

Lack of strict adherence to The Three Rules is the same. But since there are only Three Rules, and there are so many wonderful things to eat that are within The Rules, it can be done. It is hard. Do it anyway.

Mind Tricks And Mantras

I have mentioned many techniques that have helped me and my patients stick to The Rules. You can think of junk food (bad carbs) as a dangerous drug or addictive activity to help you avoid eating a treat at work. You can think of cheating on The Rules as cheating on a spouse. I often call them mind tricks, but trick may not be the right word. They are motivational techniques to accomplish the task at hand. Another technique is to think only of today, as if today is all there is. Don't forget, the present really is all we know for sure that we have. When you are working on a diet plan or any positive change in your life, it is daunting if you think in terms of years, months, or even days. Patients ask me, "Do I need to do this forever?" First, you don't need to do anything, you can just go on with whatever problem you are trying to improve. But I say, "No, you just don't eat junk food today." You only follow The Rules today. When tomorrow comes, you say the same thing. All we have is today, so eat healthy today. This is the exact opposite of what we usually do when we are eating junk food. We say that we will only eat it today, and then we do it for days on end. What I want you to accomplish is to eat well today. Tomorrow, another day, you do the same thing.

Any mental technique or mind trick you can use is good. You will know what works for you. I use mantras—words or statements that you repeat for motivation, relaxation or other areas of self-improvement. I use a few to help me relax in a tough situation and to motivate myself to accomplish a difficult task. When especially challenged, I use the phrase, "The Obstacle Is the Way," from the book I have mentioned before. Another favorite is "It is hard, do it anyway." When everyone is eating a bagel and lox, you might see me mouthing, "Do it anyway."

None of these techniques are magic. They will not cure a serious addiction and may not make you a concert pianist. But mind tricks and mantras can get you through a moment of weakness. When a tray of cookies is passed your way, picturing heroin syringes may help you say "No, thanks." When at a restaurant, repeating a mantra may help you order the caesar salad with chicken rather than the burger and fries.

Find Foods You Like

This is the fun part. When you start any diet or healthy lifestyle, you have to give something up. If you are cutting calories, you give up some high-calorie foods you enjoy. On The Three Rules, you give up foods with bad carbs. Since these foods make up much of the American diet, and you have a weight problem yourself, you were probably eating some junk food each day. It can be difficult to think of what you will eat in the future. As I have mentioned, I am frequently asked, "So what do you eat?" Fortunately, even though Americans eat a lot, junk food makes up a minimal amount of all the food options we have.

I suggest that today you go to a standard grocery store. You do not need to go to a fancy boutique store or Whole Foods, though that is fine too. Just walk up and down every aisle and look around. Most of the produce area is within The Rules, and many of the fruits and vegetables may be unknown to you. Write down things to look up later, or look them up right away on a smartphone. (I have been doing this for a while and still need to look up many of the fruits and vegetables.) You will find many recipes and techniques that are simple and tasty.

Skip the bakery. Most of the cheese and dairy section is great. I would predict there are at least 20 cheeses you have never tried. The entire meat and seafood section, excluding a few of the prepared foods, is perfect for you. Learn about anything you are not familiar with. The frozen food section is hit or miss. The potato aisle is off limits, but there are usually a few freezers of frozen vegetables worth looking at. The refrigerators have many excellent choices, some prepared, some not. You may find pickles, sauerkraut, tofu, yogurt and other healthy items here. Write down anything you haven't tried before and read about them.

It is often said we should avoid the center aisles of the store, but the Asian and international aisles usually have some excellent choices, and you should definitely check out the spices. Canned fruit is usually no good because of added sugar, but there are some canned vegetables, beans, and tomato products that are great.

Hopefully, with a walk through the grocery store, you will find dozens of foods you haven't thought of eating in a while or have never heard of. Go online or get a book and read about how to make meals within The Rules. Since this is the first book on The Three Rules, the only thing you will find online if you search for it is my site, www.TheThree-RulesToLoseWeight.com. You can also search for "low carbohydrate recipes," and "keto diet recipes," for ideas. Not every recipe on these sites will be within The Three Rules, but many will be, and you can easily modify most recipes to suit The Rules.

Do not be afraid to experiment. I have no training in cooking, other than what I learned from my mother-in-law, my wife, books, and the internet. I can only remember one meal I have ever made that was impossible for me to eat. (Without reading any instructions, I made a sauce thickened with psyllium. It had the consistency of mucus, so we threw the dinner out.) If you make mistakes, learn from them and try again. I suggest you create a file or computer database of recipes you like and make them often. You will discover that you can vary the recipes on your own. Most meat recipes will work with chicken, fish, steak, or pork with a few changes. Variations in spices will give you even more options. Will you be able to appear on a food television show? I doubt it, but you will enjoy food, accomplish something on your own, and lose weight.

The key to any lifestyle change or diet is to enjoy it. You will quit if you don't. I promise that you can enjoy eating. I promise there are foods out there that are good. I cannot imagine you not liking at least three of the dishes we served last Christmas. Like we learned as kids, sometimes, you have to try things a few times before you can say you truly like or dislike it. It took me a couple times to love hummus and guacamole. Roasted brussels sprouts were not even on my radar before I changed to a healthy diet. I never thought of roasting bell peppers in the oven or zucchini on the stove. Prepared correctly, with the right sauces and spices, these foods are wonderful. If you don't want to make food at home, it is more difficult, but most restaurants have menu items on the Three Rules. They will usually make modifications to accommodate you.

I enjoy eating. I believe you will enjoy eating more than you do now, once you have embraced The Three Rules, because you will know it is good for you, and that you are accomplishing your goals. Right now is the hard part because you are just starting. Enjoying eating is the fun part, and it will come automatically in less time than you can imagine.

Restaurants

Restaurants and takeout establishments make it more difficult to follow any diet, including The Three Rules. We discussed the basics. Order foods that follow The Rules, taking care to ask what is in everything you eat. Planning is important. I always look at the menu online, before I go anywhere to eat. If there is absolutely nothing on the menu, then I don't go there. If I have to go, then I eat at home before or after the meal. But you can usually find an entrée or even an appetizer, salad, or soup that has nothing in it that is against The Rules. Don't worry about upsetting the waitstaff. Just order what you want. If there is one side dish within The Rules, get that and eat more when you get home. Or ask for them to make it into an entrée. Or get two of them. But again, there are usually one or two items within The Rules. Get those and you are set.

My feeling is that there are many choices of restaurants to go to. Don't hide your weight loss plan from your friends and family. If they ask you if you want to go to a pizza place, tell them no. You would rather go to a different restaurant with choices for you, that may also have pizza for them to order. If they want food with bad carbs, most restaurants can accommodate them. Find a restaurant that has what you want. Much more often than not, all your friends and family will also find what they want.

Enjoy Eating

Most people who get in the habit of eating junk food do not actually enjoy eating. We get so used to eating it, that we do not enjoy it. Then we often feel guilty, leading to the spiral of weight gain. I see patients who admit to eating fast food every day. I can easily see that they are not happy about it, and it always embarrasses them to admit it. I would bet that if they ate healthy, and every few weeks had a Big Mac and fries, they would enjoy that meal much more. You likely won't do well in the long run if you eat fast food once in a while, because of the All or None issue, but at least you won't be as bad off as eating it every day.

We should try to enjoy every meal. A well-prepared simple chicken dinner with roasted vegetables is tasty. You do not need fancy foods or a high-priced restaurant to make eating fun. We are not talking about stale bread and gruel. If you do not think about what you eat, just grabbing the easy takeout, I believe you are missing out on the enjoyment of healthy, well-prepared meals. When eating with intent, eating healthy, thinking about meal preparation, you will love eating much more than you may have in the past, when you were probably eating bad carbs every day.

Plateaus Or Regaining

After initial success, you may reach a plateau, where you no longer are losing weight. You might even start to gain weight. Weight gain is more common after reaching your target, when you are trying to keep it off. In nearly every single case I have seen, in myself or in others, it is caused by eating some things against The Rules. It is occasionally obvious, like eating a bagel a few days a week. But sometimes, it is subtle. The most common culprits are sauces with sugar or food additives, dressings, snack foods with processed carbs, or restaurants where the ingredients are unknown.

What I recommend you do if this happens is examine every single thing you eat or drink. (You should do this anyway, but if you are not losing weight, double your efforts.) Write down everything you eat and either confirm on the label what the ingredients are, or go online and do a search. If there is nothing there that is against The Rules, then look closely at the fruits and vegetables. If there are any possibly starchy ones, stop eating them. If you are drinking smoothies and you are not absolutely certain of the ingredients—no additives, no sugars—stop them.

I have yet to see a single failure where 100% of all food and drink consumed was within The Rules. If you have written everything down for two weeks, and you are certain that nothing you ate or drank is against The Rules, please get me a message. I would like to record the first example that I have seen where The Three Rules broke down.

Parties And Other People's Homes

When you are at someone else's home for a party, take the same care you do at a restaurant, though it is easier. There are usually many choices of food, and no one really notices or cares what you eat. You can easily find enough food within The Rules. If you are not sure, ask. That may make you uncomfortable at first, but think of it this way. Any host of a party wants you to be happy and comfortable with the food you eat. When the host is a close friend or family member, they probably already know about your Rules. This is another reason I recommend being open with your loved ones regarding your plans. My family knows I don't eat bad carbs and I don't drink alcohol. They generally have a few excellent food choices, and they don't offer me an alcoholic drink.

A helpful idea is to think like a vegan. A vegan has no trouble asking the host of a party or a restaurant's waitstaff what is in everything being served. You can easily point out your preferences, so you do not offend anyone. There are also many medical conditions that require a change in diet—allergy, diabetes, hypertension, heart disease, alcohol dependence—if you add obesity to that list, then it should not prevent us from asking anyone what is in the food they offer us.

Gifts

We all receive many gifts of food. It is common for me to get wine, candy, cookies, and other wonderful treats each Christmas. As more and more patients learn about The Rules, I receive fewer and fewer such gifts. I always thank my patients who are so generous, and if I know them well, I tell them about my habits and how my family or office staff will love them. Just like hosts at a party, everyone who gives a gift wants the recipient to be happy with it. When they realize I won't be eating the cookies, sure, there may be a brief period of awkwardness. But lying to them by telling them how I will enjoy eating it is not the right thing to do. The gift-giver would be appropriately upset with me down the road if they learned the truth.

One side benefit of receiving such a gift, one that I won't eat, is that I can give it away. I use a technique recommended in *Don't Sweat The Small Stuff,* by Richard Carlson. I give the treat to someone else, usually in my office, and I don't tell anyone, not even the new recipient of the gift. I just leave it on their desk with an unsigned note. Everyone is happy.

Office Treats

You can avoid office treats just like junk food at parties and bad-carb gifts. Just don't eat them. The most important first step is to avoid even seeing them. During the holiday season, most of the treats may be kept in a break room. Try not to go in there at all, similar to not keeping junk food in the home. If you are tempted to eat the office treats, think about whether you would use heroin, cigarettes, or other harmful things just because they were free and available. Junk food is not immediately risky, like drugs, but it will ruin your plans and damage your health in the long run. If it helps to think of heroin or cigarettes when you see an office treat, then do it. It may still be hard to avoid the treats. Do it anyway.

Travel

Travel is a challenge. You will usually not have a kitchen to make your own foods. You will eat at restaurants, with friends, family, and business colleagues. At restaurants apply what we have already talked about. If you are going on a vacation for a lengthy period in a single location, vacation rentals are great. Putting aside the other benefits of privacy, space, and cost, there are also kitchens, so you can prepare any meals you want. I just mentioned that cooking is only a chore if you decide it is. I find it fun to make a dinner with family and friends on vacation. You will also save a lot of money. If it is a ten-day trip and you avoid even a few restaurant meals, you can save hundreds of dollars.

A common theme in this book and something I talk about every day at work is licensing. We license ourselves to eat junk food on vacation, during holidays, when having an unpleasant day, and when celebrating something. It makes little sense, though.

We can always find a reason to eat junk food. Yet we have decided not to smoke, do drugs, or cheat on our spouse, simply because it is a vacation. Many people laugh when I say this. But I am serious. I ask them why they are laughing? Why is it different? We "cheat" on our diet on vacation and do not "cheat" on our spouse or use drugs on vacation because we consider cheating on our spouse and using drugs to be important to avoid at all times, even on vacation. We consider our eating habits to be flexible. But a great number of people die each year from obesity. Eating habits kill many people. I treat my diet as an important part of my life and well-being. Don't cheat yourself just because you are on vacation.

Holidays

Holidays are a significant stumbling block for many people trying to control their weight. The holiday season starts with Thanksgiving and often continues through New Year's Day and beyond. In a study in a major medical journal, it was shown that the average person gains just under a pound during the holiday season, and 20% of people gained between two and four pounds.[27] That small amount will add up over the years, but that is not the biggest problem. The holiday season derails diets. We may be partway into a few months of healthy eating, we hit November, and that is the end of it. We have a treat or two, then we eat cookies, candy, pie, and everything else.

This is where everything we just talked about becomes even more important. The All or None approach works for everyone. If you never have the first peanut butter blossom cookie, you can never have the sec-

---

[27] Yanovski, J. A., et al (2000). A Prospective Study of Holiday Weight Gain. *New England Journal of Medicine*, *342*(12), 861–867. https://doi.org/10.1056/nejm200003233421206

ond. It is hard saying no to the first one. Do it anyway. It is nearly impossible for most of us to say no to the second. Ideally, you would never be around these wonderful treats, and it is one of the few times of year where I have bad carbs in the house. This year, my wife made blossom cookies, toffee, and chocolate-butterscotch haystacks. I know myself. I could not have a single one, or I would have mindlessly gorged on all of them. It was hard.

If you want to be healthy, lose weight, and keep it off, do not have the first holiday treat. If you can see the treats in your home and can abstain, then great. In the past, I could not do it. Do not be afraid to put up measures to avoid seeing the treats. Do not keep the food in the home, or find another way not to see it.

Cheat Days

You may think my editor made a mistake, with two sections of the book being about cheat days. This redundant passage is intentional, since I feel so strongly about it. A cheat day, as you know, is a day you allow yourself to "cheat" on a diet. If you are on a low-calorie diet, you could gorge for one day. If you are on a carbohydrate-based diet, you could eat fettuccine alfredo or Oreo cookies. I do not recommend a cheat day. As I said earlier, I don't like the word "cheat." It implies you are somehow cheating the diet. No, you are cheating yourself. If it is the way you want to eat and want to live, then it is the way to eat and live every day. With The Three Rules, a cheat day removes perhaps the most important part of the plan, All or None. A cheat day too often leads to repeated, more frequent breaking of The Rules.

Why do you not have a cheat day for your spouse? Why is an alcoholic not advised to have whiskey every other Thursday? Why is a gambling addict not supposed to play blackjack in Las Vegas on his birthday? Just as one whiskey often leads to six and one hand of blackjack leads to hours of losses, one day of junk food leads to weight gain. All of your efforts are wasted. The simple fact is that an alcoholic cannot stop at one drink. If we could stop with one cheat day, we would not have a weight problem.

Saboteurs

Saboteurs are people who intentionally or unintentionally hinder your diet plan. It is unlikely that you have friends who consciously want you to fail. But you will run into those who make it more difficult for you. In the home, they will bring treats, bagels (which are treats in my family), and other junk food. In the office, they will bring treats or invite you to lunch at a place with only junk food. At a party or restaurant, they will keep asking you to try some appetizer or dessert.

We have discussed how to handle gifts and similar temptations to stray from The Rules. Sometimes the saboteur is more aggressive. They may openly tell you that you are being too restrictive, that you have to "live a little." I used to say and I still sometimes think, "I want to live a lot longer, so I eat this way." I don't recommend that. I recommend, "No, thanks." If they persist, say it again. If they persist, I recommend, "This is the way I live. I feel it is the best for me."

That usually ends it. If they keep pressing you, then they may not be the friend you thought they were. You might consider a longer conversation or even distancing yourself from them. If they push you this hard, then there could be more animosity than you think, and you are unlikely to have a good relationship in the future. Alternatively, if you think their behavior is motivated by something within themselves, low self-esteem perhaps, you could try to help them work on it. You could even ask them to join you in your weight goals, because they may have the same problem and may be envious of your strength in dealing with it.

What If (When) You Slip Up?

It is rare that someone embarks on any plan and never makes a mistake. Most reformed alcoholics slip a few times. The same is true with The Three Rules. Over the years, I have slipped more than a few times. Whether you succeed after a lapse depends on what you do next. I learned from *The Willpower Instinct* that we should imagine the failure so we will have a plan in place. I do that myself and recommend it to patients. If you have a plan for what to do, you are less likely to feel bad about yourself after the slip-up, and feeling bad leads to eating unhealthy foods. Make a plan and state it plainly. "If I eat something against The Rules, I will…" My plan is always to start again the moment I finish. I do not wait until the following day. Then it is too easy to extend the mistake for days on end. If I am back on The Rules immediately, when I wake up in the morning, I feel good about myself for having made only the one mistake. There is less risk of the snowball effect of guilt followed by more eating. Try your hardest to follow The Rules. If you do not intend to eat a treat, but eat it anyway, then follow your plan and get right back to The Rules.

Conclusion and Final Thoughts

Today is the best day to start anything.

The Three Rules to Lose Weight and Keep It Off Forever will help you control your weight. But it will be you who does the work. It will be you who learns and becomes a better person for it. It takes hard work. You can do it anyway. Do not start on this or any plan unless you are ready to commit to it, ready to do the work it takes, ready to follow through.

Experts talk about the importance of changing your lifestyle rather than starting a diet. I would alter that slightly to changing the way you live. Eat with intent, choosing whether you want to continue eating whatever you like rather than eating what is good for your life. If it is worth eating only healthy foods, it is worth eating that way every day, like brushing your teeth, showering, and not smoking. Over the years, I have often heard patients tell me they do not smoke or drink, and when I ask them when they quit, they say, "today." I used to laugh. But really, that is all it is. Quit eating junk food today. Eat with intent starting today. Tomorrow, do the same thing. Then you are done.

We should do everything important with intent, thinking about whether it is the right thing for our lives. Whether you eat a cupcake on any given day seems too minor to think about in these terms, but that is how life is. It is made up of choices and decisions that we make right now. We are living right now, not in the future, and not in the past.

There are many things in our lives, most things in fact, that we cannot control. I will never have a full head of hair, play basketball well, remember everything I read, be a surgeon or a concert pianist. I can only control my mind and how I act in a situation. I can control my temper when someone cuts me off in traffic. I can smile when I meet a stranger. I can study to become a better physician. I can abstain from alcohol. I can exercise regularly. And I can control what I eat today.

The Serenity Prayer has existed in various forms for generations. We pray or ask for the serenity to accept the things we cannot change, the courage to change the things we can, and the wisdom to know the difference. We should try to apply this message to every day of our lives, including our health and how we eat. As it applies to losing weight and keeping it off, it is straightforward. You have the wisdom to know that you can lose weight, because all it takes is to give up bad carbs and junk food. It takes courage to make the change and give these foods up forever, and I believe you have that courage. I know that if you make the commitment, starting now, you will succeed. You will lose weight and change your life forever.

About the Author

———————○———————

Harold Oster is an internist, practicing in Plymouth, Minnesota. He went to Medical School in Miami, Florida, did his residency in San Diego, and went back to Miami to study Infectious Diseases. Currently, Dr. Oster primarily treats common medical problems in the office. Given his propensity to gain weight himself, he has taken an interest in obesity and weight management. You can visit his website at ActWithIntent.com

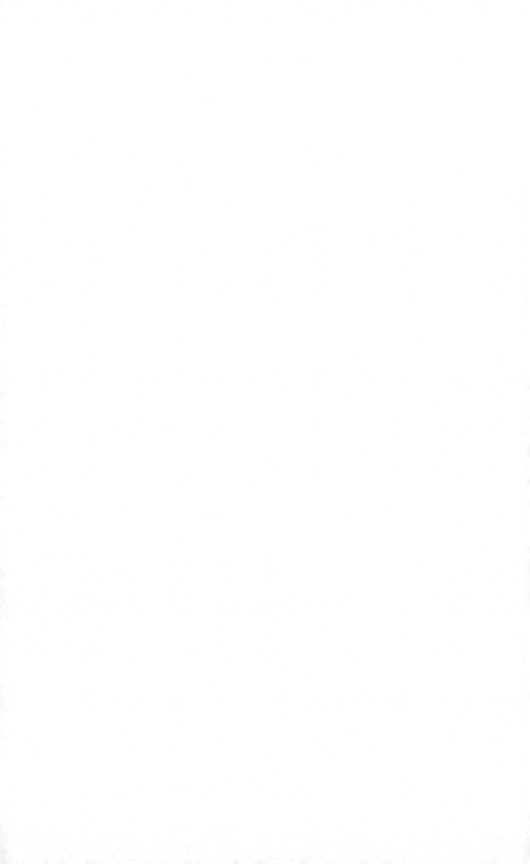

Made in the USA
Monee, IL
27 September 2021